Neurology

(CLINICAL CASES UNCOVERED)

D0541330

WITHDRAWN
FROM LIBRARY

WITHDRAWN
FROM LIBRARY

Neurology
CLINICAL CASES UNCOVERED

Malcolm Macleod
BSc (Hons), MBChB, PhD, FRCPEdin
Reader and Head of Experimental
Neuroscience, Centre for Clinical Brain
Sciences, University of Edinburgh, UK
Honorary Consultant Neurologist and
Clinical Lead for Neurology, NHS Forth
Valley, Stirling, UK

Suvankar Pal
BSc(Hons), MBBS(Distinction), MRCP, MD(Res)
Neurology Registrar, Department of Clinical
Neurosciences, Western General Hospital,
Edinburgh, UK

Marion Simpson
BSc(Hons), MBChB(Hons), MRCP
Neurology Registrar, Department of
Neurology, The Austin Hospital, Melbourne,
Australia

WILEY-BLACKWELL
A John Wiley & Sons, Ltd., Publication

This edition first published 2011, © 2011 by Malcolm Macleod, Marion Simpson, Suvankar Pal

Blackwell Publishing was acquired by John Wiley & Sons in February 2007. Blackwell's publishing program has been merged with Wiley's global Scientific, Technical and Medical business to form Wiley-Blackwell.

Registered office: John Wiley & Sons Ltd, The Atrium, Southern Gate, Chichester, West Sussex, PO19 8SQ, UK

Editorial offices: 9600 Garsington Road, Oxford, OX4 2DQ, UK
                        The Atrium, Southern Gate, Chichester, West Sussex, PO19 8SQ, UK
                        111 River Street, Hoboken, NJ 07030-5774, USA

For details of our global editorial offices, for customer services and for information about how to apply for permission to reuse the copyright material in this book please see our website at www.wiley.com/wiley-blackwell

Library of Congress Cataloging-in-Publication Data

Macleod, Malcolm, Ph. D.
 Neurology / Malcolm Macleod, Marion Simpson, Suvankar Pal.
   p. ; cm. – (Clinical cases uncovered)
 Includes bibliographical references and index.
 ISBN 978-1-4051-6220-3
 1. Nervous system–Diseases–Problems, exercises, etc.   2. Nervous system–Diseases–Case studies.   3. Neurology–Problems, exercises, etc.   4. Neurology–Case studies.   I. Simpson, Marion.   II. Pal, Suvankar.   III. Title.   IV. Series: Clinical cases uncovered.
   [DNLM: 1. Nervous System Diseases–Case Reports.   2. Nervous System Diseases–Problems and Exercises. WL 18.2 M165n 2011]
 RC343.5.M28 2011
 616.8–dc22
                                                              2010024552

A catalogue record for this book is available from the British Library.

Set in Minion 9 on 12pt by Toppan Best-set Premedia Limited

Printed and bound in Singapore by Markono Print Media Pte Ltd

2   2011

Contents

(Part 3) **Self-assessment, 124**

Preface

This book has been written by three neurologists who (we hope!) are nearer the beginning of our careers than the end, and at the time of writing two were still in formal neurological training. Our intention is to give the reader a new perspective to understand better what the phenomenal advances in our understanding of the brain mean in day to day clinical practice. In the past such books existed as the major medium through which factual knowledge was communicated to medical students and clinicians. However, such has been the pace of scientific discovery, that role has for some time been obsolete. More recently, textbooks found a role in providing research syntheses, bringing together primary evidence to give recommendations for diagnosis and management. However, with the growth of systematic tools to provide unbiased and timely research synthesis (such as used by the Cochrane Collaboration), that role too is now obsolete.

But reports of the death of the textbook have been exaggerated. At its best, clinical medicine brings the fruits of scientific research to the bedside. That requires not just a knowledge of scientific facts, but an understanding of how these inform disease processes, therapeutics, and how they can help you better understand the patient in front of you. Neurological conditions such as headache, stroke, epilepsy and dementia contribute to considerable morbidity, accounting for a large proportion of presentations to doctors in both primary and secondary care. Medical students find neurological assessment of patients notoriously daunting and this 'neurophobia' persists throughout postgraduate training. Our purpose here is to show how a patient's journey can be informed by both scientific and clinical knowledge. In doing so, we use illustrative cases which, taken together, provide broad coverage of neurological conditions commonly encountered in clinical practice.

The book is organized in three parts. Part 1 deals with the basic scientific principles underlying neurological disease, and with the fundamentals of neurology history-taking and examination. Part 2 provides 27 clinical cases covering a range of neurological conditions. The sequence of these cases has been determined by formal randomisation, and so the reader may either start at the beginning or dip in and out. Some students may wish to use a particular chapter to 'walk them through' the presentation of a patient seen in clinic or on the wards. Each case is presented in sequence, with initial presentation, followed by a discussion of the key features to elicit on history and then on examination; discussion of the implications of evidence collected; appropriate investigations and the implications of findings; and management options. Each case ends with a case review and listing of key points and references. Part 3 provides plentiful self-assessment material including multiple choice questions, extended choice questions and self-assessment questions.

The book is designed for medical students with clinical attachments in neurology and in the run up to examinations. However, it will also be useful to junior doctors who are faced with patients with neurological conditions and to those undertaking further training in internal medicine, geriatric medicine or neurology. We hope that you find this book both useful and interesting, and we hope it conveys some idea of how stimulating and rewarding neurology can be.

Malcolm Macleod
Marion Simpson
Suvankar Pal

Acknowledgements

We wish to acknowledge the contribution of those who have taught us what we know about neurology and neuroscience; the mentors and teachers who have encouraged, cajoled and educated us over the years. Our colleagues in neurology, neurosurgery, neuropathology and neuroradiology have broadened our perspective on disease. The other health professionals with whom it has been a pleasure to work, in particular the nursing staff and specialist nursing staff, have taught us of the realities of life with a chronic neurological condition. Foremost among our teachers are the patients who, through their symptoms and signs, their diseases and their reactions to adversity, have educated us more than a library of books. We hope to have distilled some of that education into this book. The errors that remain are our own.

Writing this book has taken longer than we promised ourselves, our families and our publisher. We are especially grateful to Lindsay, Calum and Magnus, to Richie and to Lynn for their love and support. At Wiley-Blackwell we would like to thank Martin Sugden for the opportunity to write the book, to Karen Moore and to Laura Murphy for sticking with us until the end. Particular thanks are due to Rustam al Shahi Salman and Will Whiteley for helpful discussions and input to the early development of the book.

We would like to acknowledge the Department of Neuroradiology, Western General Hospital, Edinburgh for the provision of some of the radiological images. MM is especially grateful to Judi Clark, Steph Fleming and Carole Condie for their administrative support.

How to use this book

Clinical Cases Uncovered (CCU) books are carefully designed to help supplement your clinical experience and assist with refreshing your memory when revising. Each book is divided into three sections: Part 1, Basics; Part 2, Cases; and Part 3, Self-assessment.

Part 1 gives you a quick reminder of the basic science, history and examination, and key diagnoses in the area. Part 2 contains many of the clinical presentations you would expect to see on the wards or crop up in exams, with questions and answers leading you through each case. New information, such as test results, is revealed as events unfold and each case concludes with a handy case summary explaining the key points. Part 3 allows you to test your learning with several question styles (MCQs, EMQs and SAQs), each with a strong clinical focus.

Whether reading individually or working as part of a group, we hope you will enjoy using your CCU book. If you have any recommendations on how we could improve the series, please do let us know by contacting us at: medstudentuk@oxon.blackwellpublishing.com.

Disclaimer

CCU patients are designed to reflect real life, with their own reports of symptoms and concerns. Please note that all names used are entirely fictitious and any similarity to patients, alive or dead, is coincidental.

List of abbreviations

ACE	Addenbrooke's Cognitive Examination
ACE	angiotensin-converting enzyme
AD	Alzheimer's disease
ADNFLE	autosomal dominant nocturnal frontal lobe epilepsy
ALT	alanine aminotransferase
ANA	antinuclear antibody
ANCA	antinuclear cytoplasmic antibody
APTT	activated partial thromboplastin time
ASOT	antistreptolysin O titre
AST	aspartate aminotransferase
ATP	adenosine triphosphate
ATPase	adenosine triphosphatase
CI	confidence interval
CIDP	chronic inflammatory demyelinating polyradiculoneuropathy
CJD	Creutzfeldt–Jakob disease
CK	creatinine kinase
CMV	cytomegalovirus
CNS	central nervous system
COMT	catechol-O-methyl transferase
CRP	C-reactive protein
CSF	cerebrospinal fluid
CT	computed tomography
CTA	computed tomography angiography
CTS	carpal tunnel syndrome
DDAVP	deamino-D-arginine vasopressin
DNA	deoxyribonucleic acid
DSA	digital subtraction angiography
DVT	deep vein thrombosis
EBV	Epstein–Barr virus
ECG	electrocardiogram
EEG	electroencephalograph
ELISA	enzyme-linked immunosorbent assay
EMG	electromyography
ESR	erythrocyte sedimentation rate
FBC	full blood count
fMRI	functional magnetic resonance imaging
GABA	gamma-amino-butyric acid
GCS	Glasgow Coma Scale
GEFS+	generalised epilepsy febrile seizures plus
GGT	gamma-glutamyl transferase
GP	general practitioner
GPi	globus pallidus interna
GTP	guanosine triphosphate
Hb	haemoglobin
Hct	haematocrit
HD	Huntington's disease
HIV	human immunodeficiency virus
HMSN	hereditary motor and sensory neuropathies
HSV	herpes simplex virus
HTLV	human T-cell leukaemia virus
ICA	internal carotid artery
ICP	intracranial pressure
ICU	intensive care unit
IIH	idiopathic intracranial hypertension
INR	international normalised ratio
IVIG	intravenous immunoglobulin
L-DOPA	L-dihydroxy-phenylalanine
LP	lumbar puncture
MAO	monoamine oxidase
MCV	mean corpuscular volume
MMSE	Mini-Mental State Examination
MND	motor neuron disease
MRA	magnetic resonance angiography
MRI	magnetic resonance imaging
MRV	magnetic resonance venography
MS	multiple sclerosis
NCS	nerve conduction study/ies
NMDA	N-methyl-D-aspartate
NMO	neuromyelitis optica
NNT	number needed to treat
NSAIDs	non-steroidal anti-inflammatory drugs
PCR	polymerase chain reaction
PD	Parkinson's disease
PEG	percutaneous endoscopic gastrostomy
PET	positron emission tomography
RR	relative risk

SAH	subarachnoid haemorrhage		TFT	thyroid function test
SIADH	syndrome of inappropriate antidiuretic hormone secretion		TIA	transient ischaemic attack
			tPA	tissue plasminogen activator
SLE	systemic lupus erythematosus		U&E	urea and electrolytes
SNr	substantia nigra pars reticulata		WCC	white cell count
TACS	total anterior circulation syndrome			

Basic science

The human nervous system is one of the most intricate of all bodily organs and new insights into its structure and function over recent decades have gone only part of the way towards unravelling the mysteries of this complex computer. The system is easiest to understand when broken down into manageable parts. Both the central and peripheral nervous systems are composed of nerve cells or neurons, which are organised in networks and serve various functions.

The processes underpinning these functions are complex, and can go wrong in lots of different ways. Much of the functioning, and malfunctioning, of the brain remains closed to us, and research continues apace. However, we are now gaining insights across a range of neurological diseases of the fundamental mechanisms that cause those diseases, and these are reviewed here. Of course, as information marches on some of what follows may prove to be at best an approximation of biological truth; but it is a better, more complete approximation than has been possible at any time in the past.

Neurons and synapses

Neurons are shaped like a tree, with a cell body (the central part of the tree), an axon (the trunk) which conveys information from the cell body to the next nerve or muscle cell in the network, and dendrites (the roots) which receive inputs from other cells (Fig. A). The connection between two nerve cells is called a synapse, and information is transmitted between cells across synapses by chemicals called neurotransmitters. Neurons in the central nervous system are very small, but in the peripheral nervous system can transmit information across long distances; a lumbar anterior horn motor neuron axon (travelling from the lumbar region of the spinal cord to the feet) can be as long as 1 m, but only 10 μm wide. This

is the equivalent of a drinking straw (5 mm wide) that is 500 m long! A sensory nerve from the big toe ending in the post-central sensory strip of the brain could be equivalent to a drinking straw of 1 km in length.

Like cardiac myocytes, neurons are excitable cells, meaning that they rely on electrical impulses to transmit information. The electric charge of a neuron is created and maintained by a delicate balance between positively and negatively charged ions, which enter and leave the cell through channels (such as sodium and potassium channels), the opening of which is usually regulated by pumps (such as sodium–potassium ATPase) in the cell membrane. When a neuron fires, rapid changes in ions within the cell (and their associated electric charges) cause depolarisation and repolarisation of the cell.

The action potential

The various inputs to any given neuron lead to changes in the transmembrane potential in the region of the axon hillock. When the depolarisation raises the potential from the resting value (around −90 mV) to around −40 mV, specialised voltage gated sodium channels open, allowing the influx of sodium ions down their concentration gradient, with depolarisation and reversal of transmembrane potential to around +40 mV. This leads to changes in the transmembrane potential further down the neuron, and when sodium channels there sense that this has reached −40 mV they too open, and so the depolarisation is propagated down the neuron into the axon itself. In time the sodium channels close, and the resting balance of ions across the membrane is restored by sodium–potassium ATPase, a pump that consumes around two-thirds of neuronal energy expenditure.

Neuronal axons are covered in an insulating substance called myelin, which is a component of Schwann cells (in the peripheral nervous system) and oligodendrocytes (in the central nervous system). The effect of the myelin sheath is to provide insulation and allow faster conduction along the axon, as well as providing metabolic

Neurology: Clinical Cases Uncovered, 1st edition. © M. Macleod, M. Simpson and S. Pal. Published 2011 by Blackwell Publishing Ltd.

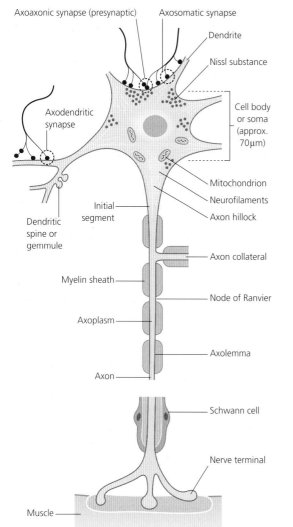

Figure A The structure of a neuron.

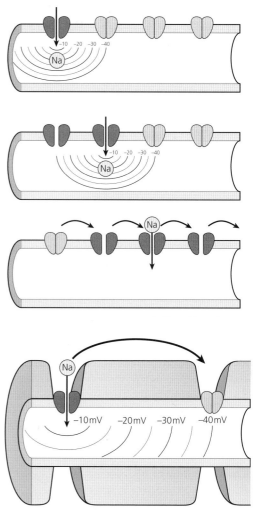

Figure B Saltatory conduction.

support for the cell. Along the course of the axon there are tiny gaps between myelinating cells called nodes of Ranvier (which are up to 2 mm apart). The action potential jumps between these nodes by a process called saltatory conduction, which speeds up the process of conduction (Fig. B).

Disorders affecting the myelin sheath are usually immune-mediated and include multiple sclerosis and Guillain–Barré syndrome. When the myelin sheath is damaged, conduction velocity along the axon is reduced and the cell may die, producing neuronal atrophy. Multiple sclerosis (MS) is a disorder of cell-mediated immunity caused by recurrent attacks on oligodendrocytes, and results in sustained impairment because of incomplete remyelination and secondary axonal

damage. Neuromyelitis optica (NMO) is a related condition with recurrent episodes of optic neuritis and spinal cord inflammation. NMO is a disorder of humoral immunity caused by antibodies to the astocyte water channel aquaporin, and the prognosis is worse than that of MS.

Guillain–Barré syndrome is a disorder of humoral immunity resulting from a (usually monophasic) attack on Schwann cells causing demyelination. Antibodies raised in response to infection such as *Campylobacter* cross react with gangliosides expressed on the surface of Schwann cells and invoke an inflammatory response. The principal effect on nerve conduction is reduced conduction velocity rather than the reduced compound action potential seen in axonal neuropathies. This reflects the fact that while the axons are usually stripped of their myelin sheath, the underlying axons seldom die off, so that conduction is slower but the number of cells contributing to the compound action potential remains relatively constant.

Synaptic transmission

Neurons generally use chemical signalling to communicate with each other and with muscles at specialised structures called synapses (or, in the case of muscles, the neuromuscular junction). When a neuron depolarises, the wave of depolarisation spreads along the axon and reaches the presynaptic terminal at the end of the axon. The resultant change in membrane potential is sensed by voltage gated calcium channels which then open, leading to the influx of calcium. The resulting increase in intracellular calcium triggers the binding and fusion of presynaptic vesicles, which contain the neurotransmitters to the presynaptic membrane, leading to the release of transmitter to the synaptic cleft. The neurotransmitters diffuse across the synaptic cleft to reach the postsynaptic membrane on the next neuron in the network (Fig. C).

There follows a rapid increase in transmitter concentration at the postsynaptic membrane. Some of this transmitter binds to receptors on the postsynaptic membrane, some undergoes re-uptake by the presynaptic nerve terminal and some is metabolised by enzymes (such as acetylcholinesterase or catechol-O-methyl transferase).

Postsynaptic receptor binding

When it reaches the postsynaptic membrane, the neurotransmitter binds to receptors which are usually proteins. There are two main types of receptor: ion channel-associated receptors and G-protein-coupled receptors. The latter are associated with G-proteins that result in the activation or inhibition of GTPases. The former are associated with ion channels (ligand gated) so that binding of the neurotransmitter to the receptor causes opening of the channel allowing influx or efflux of ions along their concentration gradient. Opening of a single ion channel could never cause sufficient ion flows to raise the intracellular potential enough to result in neuronal depolarisation, but if the summation of inputs from different ion channels at different postsynaptic membranes is sufficient, depolarisation will occur, with opening of voltage gated channels and thereby initiation of an action potential.

These same receptors are the site of action of many of the drugs used in the treatment both of neurological diseases and of other conditions. For instance, many of the clinical manifestations of Parkinson's disease are caused by degeneration of neuronal pathways between the substantia nigra and the striatum (so-called nigrostratal pathways). The neurons that are involved in abnormal degeneration in Parkinson's disease have their cell bodies in the substantia nigra ('nigra', or black, at histological examination because of the presence of the machinery needed to make dopamine) and terminate in the striatum, where the dopamine is released.

The clinical manifestations of Parkinson's disease can be alleviated, in many patients, by drugs that are given systemically and which bind to, and activate, striatal dopamine receptors. These are called dopamine agonists. Similarly, some of the more florid manifestations of schizophrenia can be ameliorated by drugs that block dopamine signalling at specific receptor subtypes, and these are called dopamine antagonists.

Drug–receptor interactions

Information about the interaction of drugs (and endogenous chemical ligands) with receptors on neurons can be used to work out how often the drug should be given and what the appropriate dose should be. The rate at which a drug binds to (or associates with) a receptor can be described by an association constant k(a), and the rate at which drug–receptor complexes break up can be described by a dissociation constant, k(d). The rates of association and dissociation depend on these constants and on the amount of ligand (L), receptor (R), and ligand–receptor (LR) complexes:

Rate of association $= k(a) \cdot [L] \cdot [R]$
Rate of dissociation $= k(d) \cdot [LR]$

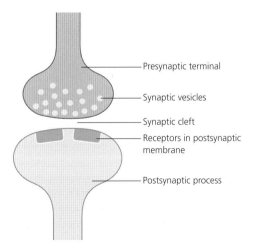

- Presynaptic terminal
- Synaptic vesicles
- Synaptic cleft
- Receptors in postsynaptic membrane
- Postsynaptic process

Figure C A synapse.

Soon after neurotransmitter release or drug delivery, an equilibrium is reached where the rates of association and dissociation are equal, and so:

$$[L] \cdot [R]/[LR] = k(d)/k(a) = K$$

The effect of a drug is manifest when it is bound to the receptor, and the amount of bound drug is:

$$[LR] = [L] \cdot [R]/K$$

Because the total amount of receptor is fixed (at least in the short term), the maximum effect of any drug is also fixed:

$$R_{tot} = [R] + [LR]$$

Therefore,

$$[LR] = ([L] \cdot ([R_{tot}] - [LR]))/K$$

Rearranging,

$$[LR] = [R_{tot}]/(1 + (K/[L]))$$

In other words, because the number of receptors for a drug or neurotransmitter does not change at a given point in time, only a certain amount of chemical can bind to the postsynaptic cell. Once the receptors are full, no more chemical can produce an effect. Therefore sequential increases in drug concentration at the active site do not result in the same increase in receptor occupancy. In fact, over the active range of drug concentrations, there is a logarithmic relationship between drug concentration and receptor occupancy (Fig. D). At higher doses, very little can be gained from increasing drug dose. This is important when escalating agonist drug doses, for instance dopamine agonists in Parkinson's disease.

However, the relationship between drug concentration and drug metabolism (and the rate at which the drug is cleared) should also be considered. For many drugs, the rate of metabolism is proportional to drug concentration (first order kinetics), so that the more drug is available, the more enzymes there are working to clear it. However, some drugs cause the induction of the enzymes responsible for their metabolism (second order kinetics, e.g. phenobarbitone and the cytochrome p450 system), and this can result in lower concentrations both of the drug and also of other drugs, or hormones, which share that pathway. Finally, for some drugs, the metabolic pathway can become saturated (zero order kinetics), such that small subsequent increases in dose lead to substantial increases in drug concentration (e.g. phenytoin) because there are not sufficient enzymes available to clear the increased dose of drug.

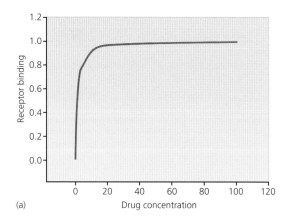

(a)

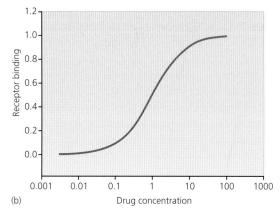

(b)

Figure D (a) Dose–response and (b) log dose–response curves.

Excitatory transmission

Neurotransmitters may be excitatory (causing the next cells in the network to become excited and fire) or inhibitory (suppressing the next cells in the network and reducing their chances of firing). The predominant excitatory neurotransmitter in the mammalian nervous system is the amino acid glutamate. Glutamate binds to a number of different receptors, some of which are linked to ion channels and others of which are coupled to G-proteins. One particular receptor deserves a special mention: the N-methyl-D-aspartate (NMDA) receptor has characteristics that allow it to fulfil special functions in information processing, but these very characteristics also make it a key player in disease states.

NMDA receptors: inward rectification

The NMDA receptor is a ligand gated ion channel. Under normal conditions, in a cell at rest, conductance through the NMDA receptor is low even when the channel is

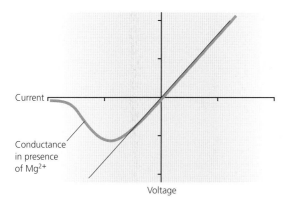

Figure E Inward rectification at the NMDA receptor.

open. This is because magnesium ions in the extracellular fluid are drawn in to the mouth of the receptor along the electrochemical gradient but are too large to pass through, so they block it. However, if the neuron becomes depolarised that electrochemical gradient is less strong, the cell is less attractive to magnesium ions, and the blockade of traffic through the ion channel is reduced, allowing other cations (predominantly calcium and sodium) to flow down their concentration gradient and enter the cell. This process is called inward rectification and can be shown in a plot of current flowing against membrane potential (Fig. E).

Long-term potentiation and memory

This property of NMDA receptors is important in the formation of memory. If a cell with several NMDA receptors is depolarised, leading to calcium and sodium influx, these ions cause the cell to remain depolarised (and therefore less attractive to magnesium ions), meaning that other ions can continue to flow into the cell for a longer period. Therefore the response of the cell to subsequent stimuli is potentiated. This phenomenon persists for some hours, and is called long-term potentiation. It provides a mechanism whereby different streams of information can be integrated, and the convergence of different signalling pathways can be recorded.

For example, imagine a set of neurons situated at the convergence of two pathways, one conveying the colour of objects and the other conveying the identification of plants (Fig. F). If different neurons receive different inputs from each of these pathways an array can be constructed. After exposure to lots of different plants, neurons receiving information on the colour 'blue' and on violets will be potentiated in response to inputs of

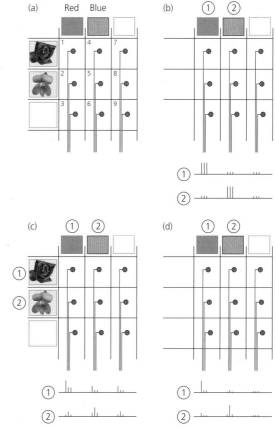

Figure F Illustration of how long term potentiation can be a substrate for memory. (a) An array of 9 neurons responds to red or blue or other colour (vertical); and to roses or violets or other flowers (horizontal). (b) Exposure to red causes activation of neurons 1–3, and exposure to violet causes activation of neurons 4–6. (c) Exposure to red and roses causes preferential activation of neuron 1, and some activation of neurons 2,3,4 and 7; Exposure to blue and violets causes preferential activation of neuron 5 and some activation of neurons 2,4,6 and 8. (d) Subsequent exposure to red causes preferential activation of neuron 1 and some activation of neurons 2 and 3; while subsequent exposure to blue cases preferential activation of neuron 5 and some activation of neurons 4 and 6. When challenged with red, neuron 1 'remembers' the rose, and when challenged with blue neuron 5 'remembers' the violet.

either 'blue' or violets, and the same will hold for those receiving information on 'red' or roses. In contrast, those capable of receiving inputs about 'blue' and roses, or 'red' and violets, will not have their inputs potentiated. So when faced with a stimulus 'rose', it is much more likely to be associated in the mind with 'red' than with 'violet'.

Excitotoxicity

As mentioned above, the NMDA receptor can also be important in disease states. The capacity for long-term potentiation and progressive increases in excitability brings with it a susceptibility to overwhelming stimulation. Where neurons are exposed to multiple, repetitive inputs over a short period (as happens during seizure activity), or where the extracellular concentration of excitatory agonists is too high for too long (as happens with failure of glial glutamate uptake) or where neurons are unable to maintain their membrane potential, then NMDA receptor channels remain open for prolonged periods, resulting in substantial rises in intracellular calcium. This in turn invokes a number of processes including activation of neuronal nitric oxide synthase, free radical production and subsequent damage to DNA, membranes and mitochondria.

If there is a failure in the delivery of oxygen or glucose to the brain (as occurs in stroke, syncope, cardiac arrest or hypoglycaemia), then neurons become unable to synthesise adenosine triphosphate (ATP), the high energy phosphate that acts as the energy source for important enzymes including sodium–potassium ATPase, and this means that action potentials can no longer occur. At intermediate levels of blood flow (e.g. syncope), or where the insult is of short duration (e.g. a transient ischaemic attack), this may have few other consequences, and neuronal viability is not impaired.

However, in the longer run the neuron must retain sufficient resources to exclude sodium (using sodium–potassium ATPase), to normalise the membrane potential, to close voltage activated channels (including the induction of voltage-dependent blocks of the NMDA receptor) and to sequester intracellular calcium. Glial cells must have sufficient energy resources to take up extracellular glutamate, or levels will rise, causing activation of the NMDA receptor. When these processes fail (e.g. in an ischaemic stroke or prolonged cardiac arrest) then neurons undergo anoxic depolarisation and swell and eventually the cell membrane will burst.

Even if the neuron is able to normalise these processes, it may be that damage incurred at the time of the insult has been such that the integrity of the cell is compromised (perhaps, for instance, through free radical-induced DNA mutations) to the extent that apoptosis occurs.

Inhibitory transmission

As well as excitatory neurotransmitters (that cause neighbouring cells to become excitable and fire), there are inhibitory neurotransmitters that suppress firing in associated cells. The major inhibitory neurotransmitter is gamma-amino-butyric acid (GABA), largely used by inhibitory interneurons. In contrast to glutamate, a major role of GABA signalling is the opening of a chloride channel, leading to influx (down a concentration gradient but against an electrostatic gradient) of chloride ions, leading in turn to hyperpolarisation of the postsynaptic membrane.

Mutations and epilepsy

Abnormalities of neurotransmitter systems are thought to be important in the pathogenesis of epilepsy and seizures. Under normal conditions, cells are prevented from firing by the inhibitory neurotransmitters, but during a seizure this inhibitory control is lost or excitatory input is overwhelming, and overactivity of the neural network results. Most brains, even in individuals without epilepsy or structural brain disease, are capable of manifesting seizure activity given a large enough insult. The Levant nut (*Cocculus indicus*) is also known as the fishberry, because when it is thrown into water the fish are stunned, float to the surface and can be easily captured; this is due to the presence of picrotoxin, a non-competitive GABA-A antagonist, which is a powerful stimulus to seizure activity. Drugs in more common use can also provoke seizures, either during acute intoxication (e.g. opiates, amphetamines) or, through the induction of tolerance, on withdrawal (e.g. alcohol).

In most patients with epilepsy the cause is not known. Some may have a history of brain injury, or of birth injury, or learning disability, or their seizures may be the consequence of a developing brain tumour. Under these circumstances, it is thought that a disruption of neuronal circuitry, and in particular of inhibitory pathways, is at fault.

Occasionally, the susceptibility to seizures can be attributed to mutations in genes encoding important regulators of neuronal excitability. For instance, mutations in the voltage gated calcium channel CaV3.2 have been found in families with idiopathic generalised epilepsy; mutations in the voltage gated sodium channel NaV1.1 have been found in families with generalised epilepsy febrile seizures plus (GEFS+); and mutations in the ligand gated nicotinic acetylcholine receptor (which has a role in modulating synaptic glutamate release) have been in found families with autosomal dominant nocturnal frontal lobe epilepsy (ADNFLE).

The neuromuscular junction

For a neural signal to result in movement of a muscle, information must be transmitted between the end of the motor neuron and the associated muscle across a specialised structure called the neuromuscular junction. When the electrical message reaches the end of the motor nerve, depolarisation of the presynaptic membrane leads to release of acetylcholine to the synaptic cleft, and this diffuses across the synaptic cleft (around 0.2 μm) to bind to nicotinic acetylcholine receptors on the muscle membrane. These are ligand gated ion channels that allow the influx of sodium and egress of potassium. The resulting increased intracellular potential is sensed by voltage-dependent calcium channels sited on the sarcoplasmic reticulum, resulting in a large increase in intracellular calcium concentrations, which in turn leads to actin–myosin crosslinking, shortening of muscle fibrils and muscle contraction.

Disorders of neuromuscular transmission

In myasthenia gravis, autoantibodies directed against the nicotinic acetylcholine receptor provide competitive inhibition, such that the degree of postsynaptic depolarisation in response to a given concentration of acetylcholine is diminished. This leads to a compensatory increase in presynaptic acetylcholine release, which may be temporarily sufficient to restore normal contractility; but in time and with repeated stimulation, presynaptic stores of acetylcholine become depleted, leading to a fatigueable weakness and a prominence of symptoms towards the end of the day. Similarly, the Lambert–Eaton myasthenic syndrome is caused by antibodies against the presynaptic voltage gated calcium channel and so inhibits presynaptic calcium entry.

Manipulation of neuromuscular transmission

Synaptic concentrations of acetylcholine can be increased by inhibitors of the enzyme responsible for its breakdown, acetylcholinesterase, and these drugs form the basis for the treatment of the myaesthenic syndromes. However, the nicotinic acetylcholine receptor has an unusual property in that sustained concentrations of acetylcholine lead to sustained channel opening and a depolarising neuromuscular blockade. As well as being the basis of the cholinergic crisis that can result from over-treatment with cholinesterase inhibitors, this phenomenon is also responsible for the action of many neuromuscular blockers used in anaesthesia, and also for the lethal effects of some chemical weapons such as SARIN.

The clinical (botulism) and therapeutic (cosmetic or antispasticity) effects of botulinum toxin are due to interference with the process through which presynaptic vesicles dock to the presynaptic membrane.

Mutations and migraine

Genetic factors can also be important in other neurological diseases. For example, familial hemiplegic migraine involves a motor aura (that is to say, unilateral loss of power rather than simply sensory change), and is caused by mutations in the pore-forming subunit of the CaV2.1 channel, the voltage gated sodium channel NaV1.1, or the a2 subunit of sodium–potassium ATPase. In transgenic animals, the calcium channel mutation causing familial hemiplegic migraine is associated with enhanced cortical spreading depression, thought to be the pathophysiological basis of migraine aura. Given the high heritability of migraine it is likely that mutations or polymorphisms in the genes encoding similar proteins are responsible for other more common forms of migraine.

Cerebral blood supply

Blood reaches the brain via two carotid arteries and two vertebral arteries. The carotid arteries divide in the neck to form Internal and external branches. The internal carotid artery enters the skull though the carotid canal to supply the brain itself. The rest of the head, including the meninges, is supplied by the external carotid artery. The middle meningeal artery enters the brain through the foramen lacerum, and is commonly damaged following head injury, resulting in the accumulation of blood between the inner surface of the skull and the dura, an extradural haematoma. No arteries cross the subdural space, but small bridging veins are present, and trauma to these causes blood to accumulate between the dura and the brain surface, known as a subdural haematoma.

The vertebral arteries join in the midline in front of the brainstem to form the basilar artery, and this divides about 5 cm later, in front of the midbrain, to form two posterior cerebral arteries. Through two posterior communicating arteries these link with the distal carotid arteries on each side, which each in turn divide to form the middle and anterior cerebral arteries. The anterior cerebral arteries are linked by the anterior communicating artery, and the anastomotic ring thus formed – the circle of Willis – ensures that occlusion of one of the major vessels in the neck does not lead to ischaemia in one-quarter of the brain (Fig. G).

However, beyond the circle of Willis arteries supply regionally defined areas with little in the way of anastomoses between these. Occlusions of the posterior, middle or anterior cerebral arteries are therefore highly likely to lead to irreversible brain injury unless reperfusion occurs.

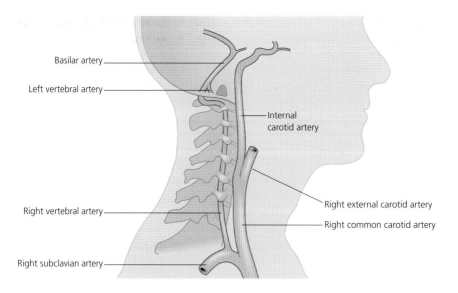

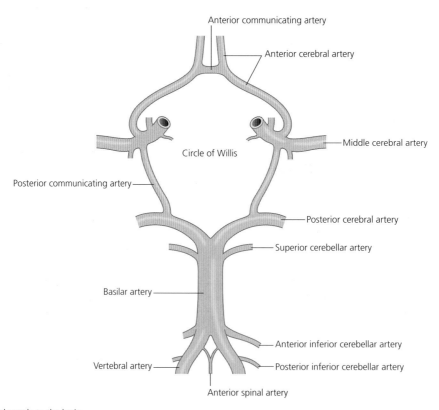

Figure G Blood supply to the brain.

Neurodegeneration

In some conditions, particular populations of neurons seem to be particularly susceptible to accelerated aging. This is probably a consequence of disruptions to processes which are unique to that population of neurons. For instance, in Parkinson's disease (PD) there is a progressive loss of tyrosine hydroxylase containing dopamine-synthesising neurons in the substantia nigra. In PD, neurons contain cytoplasmic Lewy bodies, thought to represent the accumulation of aggregates of proteins which have not been broken down in the usual way.

Around 60–80% of dopaminergic neurons are lost before the motor signs of PD become evident. The basal ganglia motor circuit consists of direct and indirect pathways and provides additional modulation to the cortical control of movement. Striatal neurons projecting to the globus pallidus and expressing D1 receptors constitute the direct pathway and those expressing D2 receptors are part of the indirect pathway. In PD, decreased striatal dopamine is held to increase inhibitory output from the globus pallidus externa/substantia nigra pars reticulata, which suppresses movement and thereby causes the clinical features of PD.

Similarly, degeneration of different neuronal populations results in the development of Huntington's disease, motor neuron disease, Alzheimer's disease, spinocerebellar ataxias and many others.

Autoimmune neurological diseases

Particular neurological dysfunctions may occur due to the presence of antibodies that bind to specific parts of the nervous system. These appear to develop because of some similarity between their intended target – an antigen on an infectious agent such as *Campylobacter* or expressed on the surface of a tumour cell – and the part of the nervous system in question. Some tumours (for instance small cell lung cancer) seem to be particularly good at provoking such responses, including a paraneoplastic cerebellar degeneration due to anti-Purkinje cell antibodies and a limbic encephalitis due to anti-voltage gated potassium channel antibodies.

CSF dynamics and idiopathic intracranial hypertension

Cerebrospinal fluid (CSF) is synthesised in the choroid plexes of the lateral ventricles and flows through the ventricular system and then to the subarachnoid space through the foramena of Luschka and Magendie of the fourth ventricle. Bathing the brain and spinal cord, CSF is reabsorbed to the blood through specialised arachnoid granulations in the walls of cerebral veins and venous sinuses.

Obstruction to the flow of CSF within the ventricular system usually occurs at the cerebral aqueduct (between the third and fourth ventricles) and results in dilation of the lateral and third ventricles and a non-communicating hydrocephalus. Where the obstruction affects the absorbtion of CSF (arachnoid granulations can become obstructed by blood following subarachnoid haemorrhage or by bacteria and inflammatory cells following meningitis), then all ventricles become dilated and this is a communicating hydrocephalus. Where CSF volume is depleted, for instance following dural puncture (post-lumbar puncture headache), spontaneous dural leak (idiopathic or spontaneous intracranial hypotension) or dehydration (as may occur after a night out), then the headache which follows is usually very positional, is better when lying flat and becomes much worse within 10 minutes of sitting or standing. Finally, in some circumstances, there appears to be an imbalance between the rates of production and absorbance of CSF. This results in raised CSF pressure, which in turn can cause pressure on the optic nerves, reduced visual fields and, if untreated, blindness. The reasons for this imbalance are not clear but may be hormonally mediated, being much more common in the overweight, in women and in those taking vitamin A preparations.

Because the spinal subdural space is in continuity with the ventricular system, CSF pressure can be measured directly at lumbar puncture. However, this should not be done where there is a non-communicating hydrocephalus, or where the presence of an intracranial mass lesion means that decompressing the lumbar CSF would rapidly establish a pressure gradient which might lead to the intracerebral contents (particularly the brainstem) being forced through the foramen magnum.

Approach to the patient

Neurology evokes fear and revulsion in a substantial proportion of medical students and junior and senior doctors. This 'neuro-phobia' is ill-founded; neurology is one of the most logical and satisfying clinical specialities, primarily because of the importance of basic history-taking and clinical skills in diagnosis and management. Revolutions in brain imaging and neurophysiology have meant that the accuracy of neurological diagnosis is increasing, and recent years have also brought about advances in therapy, so that once-untreatable conditions such as stroke and multiple sclerosis may carry a better prognosis.

The neurological history and examination are directed at answering the following questions.

1 Where is the lesion, i.e. which anatomical part of the nervous system is affected?
- Cerebral cortex
- Brainstem
- Spinal cord
- Anterior horn cell
- Nerve root/plexus
- Peripheral nerve
- Neuromuscular junction
- Muscle

2 What is the lesion, i.e. what is the most likely process causing the symptoms?
- Vascular
- Neoplastic
- Inflammatory/autoimmune
- Infectious
- Granulomatous
- Congenital
- Degenerative
- Toxic/metabolic
- Traumatic

Neurology: Clinical Cases Uncovered, 1st edition. © M. Macleod, M. Simpson and S. Pal. Published 2011 by Blackwell Publishing Ltd.

Once these two questions have been answered, the neurologist usually has a reasonable idea of the diagnosis, and can go on to arrange appropriate confirmatory investigations and consider treatment options.

History and examination

Neurological history-taking is most often the key to diagnosis. In this section, we will discuss some common neurological presenting complaints and the appropriate questions to ask in order to refine the diagnosis. The consultation should begin with a directed open question (e.g. 'Your GP has referred you here because of difficulty with your walking. Please tell me about the problem'), and followed up with a series of specific questions that aim to answer the key questions of 'where is the lesion?' and 'what is the lesion?' This is followed by a directed examination to localise the problem further within the neuraxis. This diagnostic approach can be used to evaluate any neurological symptom.

The essential principle is that the history allows the generation of various hypotheses about what might be causing the patient's symptoms; in the examination, those hypotheses are tested to allow them to be confirmed or rejected, in which case alternative hypotheses need to take their place. These refined hypotheses are then tested again by arranging investigations that might confirm or refute them. This is the so-called hypotheco-deductive approach to diagnosis. In neurology, as in so much of medicine, arranging investigations without any hypothesis about what the answer might mean is unwise.

Headache

Headache is one of the commonest reasons for referral to a neurologist. The differential diagnosis of headache can be divided as shown in Figure H.

History

A crucial part of the neurological history-taking is to identify which patients are likely to have a secondary

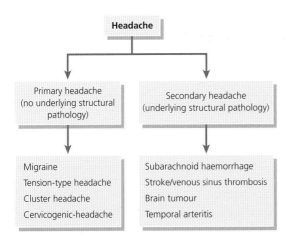

Figure H Differential diagnosis of headache.

headache (and therefore require urgent brain imaging) and which are likely to have a primary headache, which requires a different sort of treatment. The following questions are likely to be most helpful.

What is the duration of the headache?
This is perhaps the single most important question in separating primary and secondary headache. Headaches of short duration are far more likely to be secondary headaches. In general, the longer a patient has had the headache, the less likely there is to be a sinister cause.

How did it start?
Was the onset over seconds, minutes or hours? This question is important in distinguishing thunderclap headaches (the cardinal symptom of subarachnoid haemorrhage) from more benign headaches such as migraine. A thunderclap headache typically reaches its maximum intensity within seconds to minutes, and is very severe.

What is its nature?
Getting the patient to describe the pain (throbbing, dull, band-like, sharp) may give a clue as to its origin. Characteristically, migraine headaches are throbbing and tension-type headaches are band-like or dull.

Where is it?
Is it on one side or both? Is it localised to a certain part of the head? Typically migraine headaches are unilateral or more severe on one side, and cervicogenic headaches may be localised to the occipital region.

Are there any associated symptoms?
• Visual disturbance (including wavy lines and flashing lights, which are characteristic features of migraine) or visual loss (which may indicate a structural brain lesion).
• Seizures (focal or generalised) in combination with headache are highly suggestive of an underlying structural problem.
• Personality change (which may be reported by relatives rather than the patient) also raises alarm bells for a space-occupying lesion.

What makes it better?
It is important to ascertain what analgesics the patient is using, partly as a guide to the severity of the headache and its impact on their life, and partly because *analgesic overuse* is a common phenomenon particularly in primary headache syndromes, and can certainly exacerbate the existing headache. Patients with migraine typically report that analgesics alone are ineffective, and they also have to lie down in a darkened room and go to sleep until the headache passes.

What brings it on or makes it worse?
• Patients who suffer from migraine may report particular patterns or triggers, which can vary from certain foodstuffs (chocolate, cheese and coffee are common triggers) to medications (like the oral contraceptive pill) to simply changes in routine (many migraine sufferers complain of headaches on the weekend, or on the first day of a holiday when their usual routine is disrupted).
Tension headaches may be triggered or worsened by emotional stress.
• Headaches associated with raised intracranial pressure can be worsened by any Valsalva manoeuvre (e.g. coughing, bending and straining) and are characteristically worse in the morning, improving throughout the day. Typically they are relieved by simple analgesics alone.
• Headaches which are worsened by jaw movement or associated with facial pain suggest the possibility of temporal arteritis, an important cause of headache in older people (and one which is not to be missed because of its potential to threaten the sight).

Examination
Examination of headache patients is also important, noting particularly the following:

Are there any focal abnormalities on examination of the cranial nerves or limbs?

Detecting a visual field defect or hemiplegia would instantly raise the suspicion of a structural lesion as the cause of the headache.

Are there abnormalities on fundoscopy?

Detecting papilloedema would also raise alarm bells for a space-occupying lesion and would necessitate urgent brain imaging. Other causes of headache such as malignant hypertension may be associated with characteristic abnormalities on fundoscopy.

Is the blood pressure elevated?

Malignant hypertension is an important cause of headache not to be missed.

Are the temporal arteries palpable? Are they tender?

Particularly seen in elderly people, temporal arteritis is a serious cause of headache which is not to be missed as it can lead to blindness if untreated. Impalpable or tender temporal arteries raise this possibility, and an erythrocyte sedimentation rate should also be checked (although a normal value does not completely exclude the diagnosis and, if in doubt, empirical treatment with corticosteroids may be indicated).

Investigation of headache

A difficult issue is which patients with headache require brain imaging, and which modality to use. Patterns of investigation vary according to local preferences and resources. The risks of missing a serious cause of headache must be balanced against the risks of radiation, contrast allergy and the equally dangerous possibility of an 'incidentaloma' – a lesion seen on brain imaging that is unrelated to the symptoms and which may be completely asymptomatic for many years. Finding such a lesion may cause vast amounts of anxiety among patients and may lead to the performance of unnecessary invasive procedures.

As a general guide, the following groups of patients require brain imaging:

1 Any patient with headache and unexplained focal neurological signs.
2 Patients with acute ('thunderclap') headache (to exclude subarachnoid haemorrhage – may also require lumbar puncture if computed tomography (CT) scan is negative).

3 Patients older than 55 with new-onset headache.
4 Patients with systemic malignancy or immunosuppression.

Patients with the following types of headache may or may not require brain imaging:

1 Headache associated with trauma (depending on degree of trauma, conscious level and neurological signs).
2 Headache associated with symptoms of possible meningitis (in some centres it is protocol to perform lumbar puncture (LP) without CT scan; in others CT is considered mandatory before LP).

The management of headache varies according to the specific cause and is discussed in detail within the individual chapters.

Difficulty walking
History

Difficulty in walking is another common reason for referral to a neurologist and can result from lesions in various parts of the nervous system. The neurologist must ascertain the following points:

What is the time course of onset?

Was the onset *acute* (minutes to hours), *subacute* (hours to days) or *chronic* (weeks to months)? This is very helpful in distinguishing the likely underlying cause: typically, vascular diseases have an *acute* onset; inflammatory or infectious causes are most often *acute* or *subacute*; and degenerative causes are usually *chronic*.

What might be the cause of the walking difficulty?

• Motor weakness in either or both legs can cause difficulty in walking because the legs are simply unable to support the person's weight.
• Ataxia or disturbance of balance can cause difficulty walking in the absence of weakness because of unsteadiness. This can be due to a problem in the vestibular system (typically described as vertigo with or without hearing disturbance or tinnitus), in the brainstem/cerebellum (central ataxia, which may be associated with incoordination of the limbs or limb weakness on examination) or in the peripheral nervous system (called sensory ataxia, where the problem is a lack of proprioceptive information from the periphery; typically this type of ataxia is worse in the dark because there are no visual cues to guide movement).

What is the distribution of symptoms?

If motor weakness is the cause of the walking difficulty, it is important to ascertain whether one leg or both are affected, and whether there is any involvement of the arms (which places the lesion much higher up in the nervous system) or cranial nerves (which might suggest a multifocal process or a disturbance in the brainstem or even the peripheral nervous system (e.g. Guillain–Barré syndrome).

Are there any associated symptoms?

Sensory disturbance in association with motor weakness would suggest a process affecting the nerve roots or peripheral nerves. The distribution of sensory involvement (e.g. dermatomal versus glove-and-stocking) may guide the clinician further towards localisation.
• If there is motor weakness and a sensory level (described by the patient as a band-like sensation around the trunk), this is highly suggestive of a spinal cord lesion as a cause of the symptoms.
• Bowel or bladder symptoms in association with motor weakness would suggest a spinal cord lesion.
• Auditory symptoms (tinnitus or hearing loss) in association with difficulty walking may point to a disturbance of the brainstem or vestibular system.

Is the patient taking any drugs that could be causative?

The anticonvulsant phenytoin can cause ataxia. Various drugs can cause difficulty walking via a peripheral neuropathy (e.g. amiodarone, isoniazid, alcohol). Folate supplementation in the absence of B12 replacement can theoretically cause or exacerbate subacute combined degeneration of the cord.

How far can the patient walk?

This is an important functional index and can help determine the need for hospitalisation and gait aids.

Examination

The goals of the examination of a patient with walking difficulty are: (1) to attempt to localise the neurological lesion, and (2) to gain some idea of the patient's functional walking ability. The following are important points to note.

Gait

First, observe the patient (using whatever gait aids they require) looking for abnormalities of gait. In particular, look at:

• Starting off – does the patient have any hesitancy or difficulty initiating gait (a feature of Parkinsonism)?
• Do they have normal arm swing (reduced arm swing is another feature of Parkinsonism)?
• Is their stride length normal?
• Is their gait broad-based or narrow-based?
• Is there asymmetry between the two sides, signifying a hemiplegia or antalgic gait?
• Are they particularly unsteady on turning round, or does it take a long time to do so?

If the patient is able, watch them getting up out of a chair, squatting down and up, and doing heel–toe walking. Romberg's test can be performed (the patient is asked to stand steady and then close their eyes, and if they become suddenly more unsteady when the visual input is lost, the test is deemed positive and suggests a sensory ataxia with impairment of proprioception).

Cranial nerves

• Abnormal eye movements may accompany walking difficulty, for example in Wernicke's encephalopathy (ataxia, confusion and ophthalmoplegia as a result of thiamine deficiency) or in the Miller–Fisher variant of Guillain–Barré syndrome (ataxia, areflexia and ophthalmoplegia as a result of autoimmune polyneuropathy). Impaired eye movements can accompany Parkinsonism or the Parkinson's plus syndromes (e.g. progressive supranuclear palsy).
• Facial asymmetry or hemianopia may accompany a hemiplegia, which in turn can cause walking difficulty.
• Nystagmus can be a sign of cerebellar or brainstem dysfunction, or it can occur with peripheral vestibular disease, all of which can manifest as difficulty walking.

Limb examination

Examination of all four limbs is necessary, including tests of limb tone (increased tone can manifest as a spastic gait), power, coordination (looking for signs of cerebellar ataxia), sensation (particularly proprioception and light touch) and reflexes. The goal of the limb examination is to localise the problem as lower motor neuron or upper motor neuron pathology, to further direct investigations.

Visual disturbance

The evaluation of visual disturbance requires a careful history as well as an accurate neurological examination, as it can result from lesions in various parts of the nervous system (Fig. I). Table A lists some of the differential

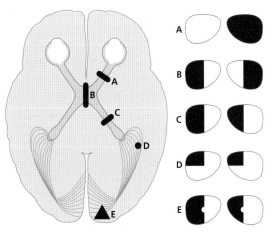

Figure I Lesions of the visual pathways. Lesions of the optic nerve (A) lead to monocular visual loss , of the optic chiasm (B) to bitemporal hemianopia, and of the optic tract (C), optic radiation or geniculostriate tract (D) or striate cortex (E) to varying degrees of homonymous hemianopia. Lesions of the optic tract cause a complete homonymous hemianopia (C), whereas those of the striate cortex, particularly if vascular, can have sparing of macular vision (E). Some fibres course inferiorly around the occipital horn of the lateral ventricle (Meyer's loop), and lesions here cause a homonymous upper quadrantanopia (D). Lesions affecting the upper, more direct fibres of the tract cause a homonymous lower quadrantanopia.

Table A Differential diagnosis of visual loss.

Monocular		Binocular	
Transient	**Persistent**	**Transient**	**Persistent**
Amaurosis fugax	Optic neuritis	Migraine	Cerebral infarction
Glaucoma	Ischaemic optic neuropathy	Visual cortical transient	in visual radiation
Visual obscurations	Retinal artery occlusion	ischaemic attack	Leber's
Retinal migraine	Retinal vein occlusion	Occipital seizure	hereditary optic
	Retinal/vitreous haemorrhage		neuropathy

diagnoses of visual loss. The following questions are important:

What is the pattern of visual disturbance?

Visual symptoms can be misleading to the patient, in that it may not be possible for them to differentiate a monoc-ular visual problem from a homonymous field defect on the same side – history and examination must be interpreted in conjunction with each other. The following are possible patterns of visual problems:

- Monocular
- Binocular
- Homonymous field defect
- Bitemporal field defect
- Central field defect

What was the time course of onset (and offset)?

As in other parts of the nervous system, a sudden onset suggests a vascular cause, and the visual pathways are vulnerable to ischaemia at various sites along their trajectory:

- Amaurosis fugax – transient monocular visual loss caused by retinal artery ischaemia, often secondary to carotid stenosis causing embolism or hypoperfusion.
- Anterior ischaemic optic neuropathy – persisting unilateral visual loss due to ischaemia of the optic disc, often secondary to temporal arteritis or atherosclerotic disease.
- Homonymous hemianopia – visual loss in the same hemifield in both eyes, usually secondary to a cerebral infarct in the contralateral hemisphere in the visual radiation. Incomplete lesions can cause a homonymous quadrantanopia.
- Cortical blindness – bilateral parieto-occipital infarcts causing visual loss accompanied by denial/confabulation.

Is there associated eye pain or redness?

Local (ophthalmological) causes of visual disturbance are often associated with eye pain and/or redness, including:

- Glaucoma
- Uveitis
- Iritis

Is there associated headache?

- Acute onset headache with visual loss may suggest serious pathology, such as a cerebral infarct or haemorrhage affecting the optic pathways.
- Migraine is commonly associated with visual symptoms, which can be visual loss but are more often 'positive symptoms' such as jagged lines or flashing lights in part of the visual field.

Does the patient have any relevant medical history?

- Vascular risk factors (e.g. hypertension, atrial fibrillation, diabetes and age) can predispose to ischaemic visual loss.

• Hypercoagulability and bleeding diathesis can predispose to retinal vein occlusion and haemorrhage, respectively.

• A history of previous transient neurological symptoms in conjunction with visual loss typical of optic neuritis may suggest a diagnosis of multiple sclerosis.

Speech disturbance

There are several speech problems that may be referred to neurologists, and it is important to be clear about the definitions of each.

• *Dysphasia*: impairment of production (expressive dysphasia) or comprehension (receptive dysphasia) of language, in either the spoken or written form. Often, patients will have a mixture of expressive and receptive dysphasia. Aphasia is a term that really means 'very severe dysphasia' (to the extent that the patient cannot speak at all) but is sometimes just used interchangeably with dysphasia.

• *Dysarthria*: impairment of articulation of words, with normal content. Very severe dysarthria is called 'anarthria' and is sometimes difficult to distinguish clinically from expressive dysphasia because the patient may not be able to produce any meaningful words at all.

• *Dysphonia*: impairment in the quality of the voice tone, leading to a hoarse or soft voice.

Speech disturbances can result from lesions in various sites of the nervous system.

Dysphasia

Dysphasia is always related to a lesion in the cerebral cortex, usually in the dominant hemisphere (the left hemisphere for most people, particularly right-handers). There is a lot of variation between individuals as to the precise location of language within the cerebral hemisphere. Classically, dysphasia is further categorised as follows:

• *Wernicke's dysphasia*: fluent expressive dysphasia (both spoken and written) with paraphasic errors (substituting words which are phonetically or semantically similar), poor naming and poor comprehension. Results from a lesion in Wernicke's area in the posterior superior temporal gyrus of the dominant hemisphere.

• *Broca's dysphasia*: non-fluent expressive dysphasia, with relatively preserved comprehension but impaired repetition and naming. Results from a lesion in Broca's area in the inferior frontal lobe.

• *Transcortical motor dysphasia*: similar to Broca's dysphasia, but with preserved repetition, resulting from a lesion in the superior frontal lobe of the dominant hemisphere.

• *Conduction dysphasia*: fluent speech and preserved comprehension, but impaired repetition and naming. Results from a lesion in the arcuate fasciculus, the site of communication between Wernicke's and Broca's areas.

Dysarthria

Dysarthria can result from lesions in the cerebral cortex (affecting the motor cortex responsible for the muscles of articulation), brainstem, lower cranial nerves (particularly the facial nerve, glossopharyngeal nerve and hypoglossal nerve), anterior horn cell, neuromuscular junction or the facial muscles themselves.

Dysphonia

Dysphonia can result from local problems with the larynx (e.g. laryngitis, trauma or laryngeal tumours), as well as neurological lesions affecting the recurrent laryngeal nerve (such as malignant infiltration from a lung cancer) or the vagus nerve (as part of a bulbar palsy, or in association with hypothyroidism or amyloidosis).

Examination

A neurologist must have a clear idea of the differences between these speech disorders and have a method of testing them which covers all aspects of speech. A suggested examination is as follows:

1 *Open with a general question* that allows you to hear the patient's spontaneously generated speech (paying attention to the quality of the sound as well as the linguistic content), for example:
  • 'What did you have for breakfast?'
2 *Test the patient's comprehension*, initially with a one-stage command, moving on to more complex commands if they get it right:
  • 'Touch your nose'
  • 'Touch your nose then close your eyes'
  • 'Touch your right ear with your left hand, point at the ceiling and then the floor'
3 *Test their ability to name objects*, and if they answer the first one correctly, try a more complicated word, for example:
  • 'Pen' and 'nib'
  • 'Watch' and 'strap'

It is often helpful to have a set of picture cards with various objects to perform a more complete test.

4 *Test articulation* (and repetition) with some tongue-twisters:

- 'West Register Street'
- 'Baby hippopotamus'
- 'British constitution'

If appropriate, you can go on to test specific skills such as reading and writing, or generation of lists of words (this is a test of executive function as well as language).

Details of the evaluation of other neurological symptoms will be presented in the forthcoming chapters. These are designed to give readers an idea of the methodological approach to history-taking in neurology.

Investigations in neurology
Brain imaging

Advances in the quality and speed of brain imaging have brought about huge developments in neurology as a speciality. The most widely used modalities include the following.

Computed tomography (CT) scan: based on X-ray technology

- *Uses*: acute stroke, subarachnoid haemorrhage, head injury, bony lesions, first test for suspected space-occupying lesion or venous sinus thrombosis.
- *Advantages*: rapid, safe for unstable or uncooperative patients, reliable for detection of blood, high resolution for examination of cerebral vasculature and bony structures.
- *Disadvantages*: radiation dose, relatively low resolution for brain parenchyma.

Magnetic resonance imaging (MRI): based on magnetic fields and radiowaves

- *Uses*: stroke (particularly diffusion-weighted imaging), demyelinating diseases and other white-matter lesions, high resolution imaging of tumours or epileptogenic lesions.
- *Advantages*: no radiation dose, high resolution, can be combined with functional MRI to assess patterns of brain activation associated with particular tasks.
- *Disadvantages*: cost, time involved, some patients may be too unwell to be left unsupervised in scanner, not as widely available, cannot be used in patient with certain metal implants (e.g. aneurysm clips, pacemakers).

Positron emission tomography (PET) scan: based on measurement of radiation emitted after injection of a radiolabelled isotope

- *Uses*: dementia (different patterns of hypometabolism in different dementing illnesses). Increasingly being used in the investigation of stroke, epilepsy and brain tumours.
- *Advantages*: unique in its ability to explore metabolic activity in different brain regions.
- *Disadvantages*: requires injection of radioisotope, cost, not widely available.

Neurophysiology

Various methods are available for measuring the function of parts of the nervous system.

Electroencephalograph (EEG)

EEGs allows recording of cerebral electrical impulses via electrodes on the scalp or sometimes implanted intracranially. May be useful in the diagnosis and characterisation of epileptic seizures (although a normal EEG does not rule out a diagnosis of epilepsy) and in particular in the diagnosis of non-convulsive status epilepticus. Also useful as an indicator of encephalopathy (such as in encephalitis, Creutzfeldt–Jakob disease (CJD) or metabolic encephalopathy) and as an adjunct to prognostication in coma or hypoxic brain injury.

Nerve conduction studies (NCS)

These are the electrophysiological measurement of conduction in various nerves. Broadly, impaired conduction may by due to axonal damage, reducing signal amplitude, or to damage to the myelin sheath, causing slowed nerve conduction. The features of these axonal and demyelinating neuropathies are discussed in Table B. Nerve conduction studies are useful in the diagnosis of neuropathies such as carpal tunnel syndrome and Guillain–Barré syndrome.

Electromyography

Electromyography is the measurement of the electrical potential (spontaneous or voluntary activity or in response to electrical stimulation) generated by muscle cells via needles inserted into the muscles. It is useful in the diagnosis of myopathies, disorders of the neuromuscular junction (e.g. myasthenia gravis) and anterior horn cell disease (e.g. motor neuron disease).

Lumbar puncture

Examination of the cerebrospinal fluid (CSF) obtained via lumbar puncture can be extremely helpful in various

Table B Features and examples of axonal and demyelinating neuropathies.

	Axonal	Demyelinating
Conduction velocity	Normal	Slow
Amplitude	Reduced	Usually normal
Distal latency	Normal	Prolonged
Examples	Diabetes	Guillain–Barré syndrome
	Alcohol	
	Toxins	Chronic inflamatory demyelinating polyneuropathy
	Porphyria	
	B12 or folate deficiency	Paraproteinaemia
		Diphtheria
	Guillain–Barré syndrome (axonal form is unusual)	Refsum's disease
		Leucodystrophies
	Paraproteinaemia	Hereditary motor and sensory neuropathies types I and III
	Hereditary motor and sensory neuropathies type II	

neurological disorders. The following parameters are measured:

• *CSF opening pressure*: this is measured using a simple plastic manometer with the patient lying on their side. If the patient was sitting upright at the time of puncture they should lie on their side before the pressure is measured. The pressure may be elevated in: idiopathic intracranial hypertension; venous sinus thrombosis; meningitis and encephalitis; following subarachnoid haemorrhage; and with markedly elevated CSF protein. CSF opening pressure may be diminished in idiopathic intracranial hypotension.

• *Protein*: elevated to varying degrees in a variety of infectious, inflammatory and neoplastic disorders of the central and peripheral nervous systems.

• *Glucose*: a low glucose level (less than 50% of serum glucose) suggests bacterial or tuberculous infiltration of the CSF.

• *White cells*: an elevated white cell count can occur in infectious, inflammatory or neoplastic conditions. Typing of white cells may be helpful (lymphocytes suggest viral infection or inflammation; neutrophils raise the suspicion of bacterial meningitis).

• *Red cells*: can result from subarachnoid haemorrhage or a traumatic lumbar puncture. Where there is doubt, testing for xanthochromia can be helpful.

• *Xanthochromia*: measurement of blood breakdown products using spectrophotometry. Positive xanthrochromia is a sign of subarachnoid haemorrhage.

• *Oligoclonal bands*: protein band patterns that are compared between CSF and serum; bands that are present in CSF alone are found in multiple sclerosis and other inflammatory diseases of the central nervous system (CNS).

• *Cytology*: useful in the detection of malignant CSF infiltration.

Biopsy

Certain conditions require biopsy of brain tissue (for the diagnosis of tumours, inflammatory conditions or cerebral vasculitis), peripheral nerve (for nerve vasculitis) or muscle (in the diagnosis of myopathy, inflammatory muscle disease or mitochondrial disease).

PART 2: CASES

Walter Jenkins, a 76-year-old, right-handed, retired chartered accountant, self-referred to the emergency department because his right hand and arm had suddenly become numb, heavy and weak.

What are the key features of the history?

1 Are his symptoms still present?
2 Did they evolve over time, or all start together?
3 What was he doing at the time his symptoms began?
4 Are there any associated symptoms?
  • Leg weakness
  • Speech disturbance
  • Headache
  • Nausea or vomiting (may suggest migraine)
  • Photophobia (dislike of light) or phonophobia (dislike of noise) (may suggest migraine)
5 Was the arm simply weak, or were there added (involuntary) movements (may suggest focal seizure)?
6 Does he have any relevant risk factors?
  • Current or previous cigarette smoking
  • Ischaemic heart disease
  • Hypertension
  • Diabetes
  • Prior history of stroke or transient ischaemic attack (TIA)
  • Recent head injury or falls
  • History of excess alcohol intake or liver disease
  • Family history of ischaemic heart disease or stroke

His symptoms developed while he was playing golf that morning at about 10.40 am. As he addressed the ball he noticed he couldn't hold the golf club correctly, and that his right hand felt strange. When he tried to explain to his

playing companion what was happening he had the greatest difficulty finding the right word. They had waited a few moments to see if things would pass, but after 5 minutes decided to head back to the clubhouse. During the walk back, which was about half a mile, he noticed that his right leg felt slightly heavy, although he had no great difficulty walking. They got back about 20 minutes after his symptoms had started, and because they showed no sign of resolution his playing partner drove him directly to hospital. As he was waiting to be assessed his symptoms began to resolve, such that when he was seen, 90 minutes after the onset of symptoms he was completely back to normal.

There had been no associated headache, nausea or vomiting, photo- or phonophobia and there were no abnormal movements in his weak hand or arm. He had previously been fit and well with no history of recent falls, had stopped smoking 30 years previously and consumed 20 units of alcohol per week. He had no history of hypertension, diabetes or recent head injury; there was no personal or family history of ischaemic heart disease or stroke.

What is the likely differential diagnosis?

He describes a transient disturbance of neurological function. The differential diagnosis lies between an attack due to focal cerebral ischaemia (a TIA), a focal seizure, a migraine aura or an attack due to some other focal disturbance of cortical function such as that seen in patients with hypoglycaemia or in association with a chronic subdural haematoma. It is important to establish the diagnosis in order to initiate appropriate treatment.

In this case, the history is most in keeping with a transient ischaemic attack, in spite of the lack of relevant risk factors. Focal seizures are usually associated with abnormal movements and with positive sensory symptomatology. The development of new migraine in a 76-year-old man would be unusual, and would usually be associated with positive sensory symptomatology and with other features such as nausea, vomiting or headache.

Neurology: Clinical Cases Uncovered, 1st edition. © M. Macleod, M. Simpson and S. Pal. Published 2011 by Blackwell Publishing Ltd.

What are the key features of the examination?

The examination should seek evidence of:

1 Continuing disturbance of neurological function:
   • Right arm or leg weakness, sensory dysfunction or reflex change
   • Speech disturbance
   • Right homonymous hemianopia
   • Facial weakness
2 Sources of thromboembolic disease:
   • Left carotid bruit
   • Atrial fibrillation
   • Valvular heart disease
3 Vascular risk:
   • Hypertension
   • Absent peripheral pulses or asymmetry of pulses
   • Obesity
   • Evidence of sequalae of diabetes (retinopathy, peripheral neuropathy, trophic ulcers)
4 Alternative diagnoses:
   • Blood sugar (by BM testing)
   • Papilloedema
   • Evidence of hepatic failure, which may indicate a bleeding diathesis

In his case he was not obese and the neurological examination was completely normal. He was in sinus rhythm with normal heart sounds, normal peripheral pulses, no carotid bruits, no evidence of the sequalae of diabetes, a BM of 6.5 mol/L and his blood pressure was 167/93 mmHg.

What is the diagnosis now?

This is almost certainly a TIA. There is nothing in the history or examination to suggest a focal seizure or a migraine, nothing to suggest an underlying structural brain lesion, no evidence of hypoglycaemia, and nothing in the history or examination to suggest a bleeding diathesis.

What is a TIA?

A transient ischaemic attack is a clinical syndrome characterised by a transient disturbance of neurological function attributed to a focal reduction in blood supply to a region of brain, not better explained by alternative pathologies, and which resolves completely within 24 hours. The causes of TIA are those of stroke, and the distinction between the two is somewhat arbitrary. Indeed, some patients with TIA have incontrovertible evidence of permanent brain injury at magnetic resonance imaging (MRI) whereas some patients with stroke have completely normal brain imaging. The prognosis for recurrence is slightly higher for minor stroke than it is for TIA, but in pathophysiological terms these diagnoses represent different severities of the same process rather than independent processes.

What investigations are required?

The focus of investigation should be to exclude alternative diagnoses and to establish if he has particular risks for recurrence. Standard chemistry will show renal function, liver function and a formal blood sugar, and cholesterol should also be tested. Full blood count will show if the platelet count is reduced (risk for haemorrhage including chronic subdural haematoma), and an erythrocyte sedimentation rate (ESR) is a useful screening test for raised intravascular inflammatory mediators such as might be seen with vasculitidies such as giant cell arteritis or with bacterial endocarditis.

Carotid dopplers will show whether he has a significant stenosis of the left internal carotid artery (Fig. 1.1), in which case carotid endarterectomy is likely to reduce his risk of recurrent stroke. He should have an ECG, and if cardiac examination is not completely normal he should also have an echocardiogram. If there is any suggestion of paroxysmal symptoms he should have a 24-hour ECG monitor to seek to capture any episodes of paroxysmal atrial fibrillation.

He should have some form of brain imaging to help further exclude other diagnoses, although in his case these will probably be normal. Where both are available, MRI is probably to be preferred over CT, and where patients present late and imaging is delayed beyond a week or so MRI is definitely superior, as it is able to detect the presence of haemorrhage after the CT signs of this have resolved.

His blood tests are all normal, with a cholesterol of 4.7 mmol/L and an ESR of 13 mm/h. Carotid dopplers showed a 75% stenosis of the left internal carotid artery (ICA). ECG, echo, 24-hour tape and a CT of the brain are all normal.

What's the big deal with him having had a TIA – he's better now isn't he?

Patients who have had one TIA are at substantial and immediate risk of recurrent TIA or, importantly, disabling stroke. This risk can be estimated using simple clinical scores such as the ADCD2 score (Box 1.1);

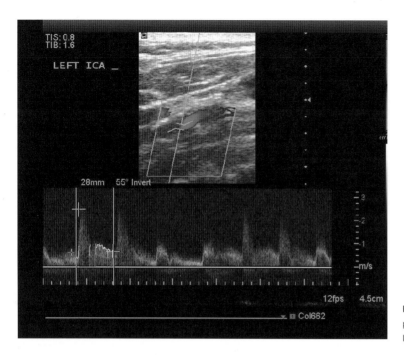

Figure 1.1 Carotid Doppler of this patient showing 75% stenosis of a left ICA.

Box 1.1 ABCD2 score

Age	>60 years	1
	<60 years	0
Blood pressure (BP)	Systolic BP > 140 or diastolic BP > 90 mmHg	1
	Normotensive	0
Clinical syndrome	Unilateral weakness	2
	Speech disturbance without weakness	1
	Neither	0
Duration of symptoms	>60 minutes	2
	10–59 minutes	1
	<10 minutes	0
History of diabetes	Yes	1
	No	0

The ABCD2 score predicts the 90-day risk of recurrent TIA or stroke

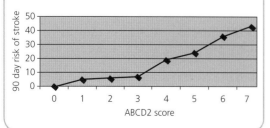

---

prompt initiation of targeted (e.g. carotid endarterectomy) or generic (e.g. antiplatelet treatment) secondary prevention measures can substantially reduce the risk of disabling stroke.

His ABCD2 score is 6 [A(1)B(1)C(2)D(2)D(0)], and therefore he is at substantial risk of recurrent stroke; he needs urgent targeted and generic secondary prevention measures to modify this risk.

How should patients with a TIA be managed?

1 *Lifestyle*: patients with a TIA may benefit from lifestyle modifications, in order to reduce the risk of further attacks. Such modifications include:
- Regular exercise
- Weight loss
- Stopping smoking
- Healthy diet

2 *Generic secondary prevention*: some measures are indicated for all patients unless there is a specific contraindication.
- Antiplatelet treatment:
  - aspirin should be started immediately, with a 300 mg loading dose followed by 75 mg/day (NNT = 67 per year)

- dipyridamole 200 mg bd, 900–1200 mg orally. While aspirin plus dipyridamole is more effective than aspirin alone the additional benefits are marginal (NNT = 125 per year), and many experts would adopt a phased approach, adding dipyridamole in patients thought to be at high risk of recurrence or in whom events occur despite being on aspirin
  - for patients who are allergic to aspirin, clopidogrel may be used as an alternative
- Cholesterol lowering treatment: statins (atorvastatin, simvastatin) reduce the risk of future vascular events, and may themselves have neuroprotective properties. They should be started immediately
- Blood pressure lowering treatment: diuretics (e.g. indapamide) and angiotensin-converting enzyme (ACE) inhibition (e.g. perindopril) reduce the risk of further vascular events and may reduce the rate of cognitive decline in patients with small vessel vascular disease

3 *Specific secondary prevention measures:*
  - In patients with atrial fibrillation, anticoagulation with, for example, warfarin reduces the risk of further stroke
  - In patients with significant narrowing of the carotid artery, carotid endarterectomy reduces the risk of ipsilateral stroke, but there is a procedural risk; the operation is of most benefit in the elderly, in men, and when performed within weeks of the index TIA or stroke. Beyond 12 weeks, the balance between risk and benefit is much less clear

Our patient is found to have a 90% stenosis of his left internal carotid artery; he is commenced on aspirin and simvastatin and referred to the vascular surgeons, who perform an uncomplicated carotid endarterectomy the following week. He is commenced on antihypertensive medication the day after his surgery, and he goes on to make an uneventful recovery.

CASE REVIEW

This 76-year-old had no vascular history or relevant risk factors, and presented with the sudden onset of weakness in the right hand and arm, developing over a few minutes and resolving completely over a couple of hours. A clinical diagnosis of TIA can be made with some confidence, and he was investigated and shown to have a tight carotid stenosis of the symptomatic side. Appropriate management of specific (carotid stenosis) and generic (antiplatelet, blood pressure, cholesterol) risk factors was instituted and will substantially reduce his risk of stroke.

KEY POINTS

- TIAs should be managed as a medical emergency because of the opportunities for highly effective secondary prevention
- The key to successful management is prompt diagnosis and investigation
- The risk of recurrence can be estimated using a simple clinical score
- Secondary prevention measures can be generic or targeted
- The benefits of carotid endarterectomy decline quickly with time

Further reading and references

Easton JD, Savers JL, Albers GW *et al.* Definition and evaluation of transient ischemic attack. *Stroke* 2009:**40**;2276–93.

Case 2 A 60-year-old man with back pain and weakness

Arthur is a 60-year-old who presents with a 2-month history of new onset back pain. He originally attributed it to the bad weather but it did not improve despite regular analgesics. When it started, he had no additional symptoms, and his GP prescribed some stronger painkillers and asked him to come back in a month if it hadn't gone away. When he returned to the GP, his pain was worse and he had great difficulty walking into the surgery; he had borrowed a friend's wheelchair to get around outside because his legs 'just wouldn't hold him any more'.

What are the key features of the history?

1 Where is the pain and does it radiate anywhere?
  • Back pain with nerve involvement may radiate down the buttocks and into the legs or feet
2 Are there any exacerbating or relieving factors?
  • Coughing, sneezing and straining may worsen pain associated with nerve root compression (radiculopathy)
3 Does he have any new symptoms of bowel or bladder dysfunction?
  • Urinary retention
  • Hesitancy
  • Frequency
  • Constipation
  • Incontinence
If present, these are extremely worrying 'red flag' symptoms which can indicate spinal cord or cauda equina compression, and require urgent attention
4 Does he have normal sensation during micturition or defaecation?
5 What is the duration of symptoms and how fast are they progressing?

  • This gives a suggestion as to the likely aetiology and may dictate the urgency with which investigations are required
6 Does he have pain, weakness or altered sensation in his legs? Does he have disturbance of balance?
7 Are there any neurological symptoms in the hands or the cranial nerves?
  • This is essential information in localising the lesion. Involvement of both hands and both legs suggests a lesion in the cervical spinal cord (or peripheral nervous system); involvement of only the legs suggests a lesion in the thoracolumbar spinal cord (or peripheral nervous system). Involvement of the cranial nerves places the lesion higher up in the brain or brainstem, or suggests a diffuse process
8 Is there a band-like sensory level around his trunk?
  • If present, this is a very strong indicator of spinal cord pathology and may help localise the site of the lesion
9 Are there any symptoms of systemic disease or risk factors for malignancy, or a history of arthritis?
  • Where cord compression is a consideration, the two most common causes are metastatic malignancy and spondylosis

Arthur reports that the pain is in the middle of his back, just below the bottom of his rib cage, and that it does not radiate anywhere else but has been becoming progressively more severe over the last month. He didn't want to come back to the doctor's early because he didn't want to take up her time. He has been constipated but he put that down to the medication, and he has been getting up several times each night to empty his bladder, although lately he has not been able to pass more than a few drops of urine and still feels that his bladder is not completely empty afterwards. His legs have felt 'heavy' for the past 10 days and over the past 2 days he has noticed some tingling in his feet on both sides. His walking has deteriorated too, and he is now able to walk only 50 m with great difficulty.

Neurology: Clinical Cases Uncovered, 1st edition. © M. Macleod, M. Simpson and S. Pal. Published 2011 by Blackwell Publishing Ltd.

He has been feeling less well in general over the last few months; he has been tired and sometimes breathless, although he put this down to his smoking habits. He used to smoke 20 cigarettes per day but gave up 2 months ago because he just didn't feel like it any more. He has lost 5 kg in weight but on systemic enquiry there are no other symptoms.

What is the differential diagnosis at this point?

> **!RED FLAG**
>
> His history is worrying because of the progressive nature of the pain and the development of leg weakness. The presence of bowel and bladder disturbance and sensory changes in the feet are also very worrying and should alert the neurologist to the possibility of spinal cord or cauda equina pathology. Given his systemic symptoms, a malignant cause is likely.

Neurological examination will help to further localise the site of the lesion. The main differential is between a lesion in the spinal cord (upper motor neuron), in the nerve roots around the cauda equina, or the peripheral nervous system (lower motor neuron), although bladder involvement would not be expected with a lesion in this area.

What are the key features of the examination?
General examination

Where malignancy is suspected, it is important to look for any clinical signs of it:
- Cachexia or signs of weight loss
- Finger clubbing
- Lympadenopathy
- Jaundice
- Pallor
- Pleural effusion or pulmonary collapse
- Abdominal masses or organomegaly
- Breast masses or axillary lymphadenopathy
- Skin lesions or rashes

Cranial nerves and upper limbs

It is important to examine both of these carefully, regardless of the fact that the complaint involves the legs, as it may change the location of the presumed neurological lesion if these are found to be abnormal.

Lower limbs

1 *Tone*: if increased, it is suggestive of an upper motor neuron lesion (although there may be flaccid weakness in the acute phase of a spinal cord injury).
2 *Power*:
   - Is there weakness, is it bilateral or symmetrical, and what is the distribution?
   - In lesions of the pyramidal tracts (i.e. the long motor pathways of the brain and spinal cord), there may be a characteristic pattern of weakness where the flexors (hip flexion, knee flexion, ankle dorsiflexion) of the legs are weaker than the extensors (hip extension, knee extension and plantar flexion). In the arms, the pattern is reversed and the extensors are weaker than the flexors
   - In lesions of the peripheral nervous system, weakness may be patchy (as in mononeuritis multiplex) or may be more marked distally (as in a length-dependent peripheral neuropathy)
3 *Coordination*: this may be abnormal as a consequence of the weakness rather than as a result of primary abnormality of the cerebellum; if there is definite weakness examining coordination may be unreliable.
4 *Sensation*: it is essential to examine sensation in the legs and trunk and to document the presence or absence of a sensory level, which can be extremely helpful if present. It is also essential to look for differences between pain/temperature (which are transmitted in the spinothalamic tracts) and vibration/proprioception/light touch (which are transmitted in the dorsal columns) as a difference in these groups of modalities might help localise a spinal lesion to a particular part of the spinal cord. It is important to map out the distribution of sensory change, and to assess whether it fits with a particular dermatome or peripheral nerve (Fig. 2.1).
5 *Reflexes*: in disease of the spinal cord (other than the acute phase where there may be flaccid weakness and areflexia), the reflexes are likely to be brisk and there may be upgoing plantars. Nerve root compression may lead to absent reflexes in the nerve involved. In diseases of the peripheral nervous system where there is demonstrable weakness on examination (indicating moderately severe nerve dysfunction), the reflexes are likely to be absent or very difficult to elicit; plantars are likely to be downgoing or equivocal.
6 *Gait*: this is useful because it gives an idea of the patient's functional status as well as helping to localise the neurological lesion.

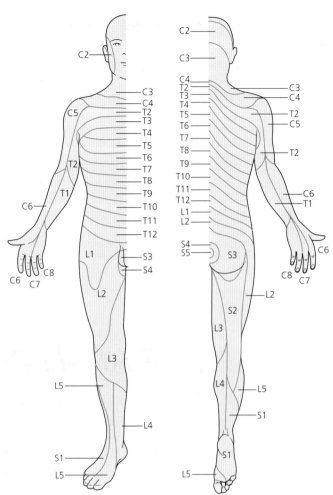

Figure 2.1 The dermatomes.

Table 2.1 Nerve roots responsible for deep tendon reflexes.

Reflex	Root
Biceps	C5, C6
Brachioradialis	C6, C5
Triceps	C6, C7
Knee	L3, L4
Ankle	S1

Table 2.1 shows the nerve roots that mediate the commonly tested deep tendon reflexes. A useful scheme for documenting the lower limb power is shown in Table 2.2.

On general examination, Arthur is thin, with sunken cheeks and his trousers are held together with a piece of string because they have become loose. His fingers are not clubbed but they are tar-stained. There is a palpable bladder but no hepatomegaly; respiratory examination is unremarkable and no skin lesions are found.

His cranial nerves and upper limbs are entirely normal. In the legs, there is no wasting or fasciculations, and tone is increased bilaterally. He has great difficulty lifting his legs off the couch, bending his knees or dorsiflexing his feet (power 3/5) and some difficulty extending his legs at the hips, straightening his legs or plantar flexing his feet (4/5). The coordination could not be tested because of this. The reflexes were brisk and symmetrical and there was clonus at the ankle bilaterally. The plantars were bilaterally and symmetrically upgoing, and there was sensory loss to all modalities up to the level of the umbilicus. On digital rectal examination there was reduced anal tone and decreased perineal sensation. He had pain on percussion of his back in the mid thoracic region.

Table 2.2 Useful scheme for documentation of limb examinations.

	Right lower limb	Left lower limb
Tone	↑↑	↑↑
Power:		
Hip flexion	3/5	3/5
Hip extension	4/5	4/5
Knee flexion	3/5	3/5
Knee extension	4/5	4/5
Ankle dorsiflexion	3/5	3/5
Plantar flexion	4/5	4/5
Great toe	3/5	3/5
Coordination	n/a	n/a
Sensation	↓ all modalities to umbilicus	↓ all modalities to umbilicus
Reflexes:		
Knee jerk	++++	++++
Ankle jerk	+++	+++
Plantar response	↑	↑

What is the most likely diagnosis now?

The history suggests a subacute onset of back pain, difficulty mobilising, leg weakness and sphincter disturbance. The signs on examination are suggestive of an upper motor neuron lesion with increased tone, a pyramidal pattern of weakness and hyperreflexia with clonus; this is the clinical picture of a spastic paraparesis (Box 2.1). The absence of any findings in the arms or cranial nerves, together with the presence of a sensory level, strongly suggest spinal cord pathology. In a patient of this age group, the most likely diagnosis would be malignant cord compression (particularly in the presence of systemic features of malignancy). Spondylitic disease is also a possibility. In any case, urgent neuroimaging is required to investigate this further.

Arthur is rushed to the radiology department for urgent imaging of his spinal cord (Fig. 2.2). This confirms the neurologist's suspicion of malignant cord compression and he is treated immediately with high-dose intravenous steroids. A chest X-ray shows a suspicious lesion and following bronchoscopy he is diagnosed with small cell carcinoma of the lung. He receives radiotherapy to the spinal cord metastasis and is commenced on chemotherapy to treat the underlying cancer. At his 3-month review he is still ambulating and is free from back pain.

Box 2.1 Causes of spastic paraparesis

- Neoplastic: metastatic tumour, intrinsic spinal cord tumour (rarely due to intracerebral parasaggital meningioma)
- Degenerative: spondylytic changes secondary to osteoarthritis
- Vascular: spinal artery infarction, haemorrhage (from spinal arteriovenous malformation or arteriovenous fistula)
- Inflammatory: demyelination secondary to multiple sclerosis or neuromyelitis optica
- Toxic and metabolic: e.g. vitamin B12 deficiency, nitrous oxide poisoning
- Infective: HIV, HTLV-1
- Hereditary: hereditary spastic paraparesis, Friedrich's ataxia

CASE REVIEW

This case describes the classic clinical picture of spinal cord compression, which is a true neurological emergency. The key 'red flag' symptoms which should alert the neurologist in this case were the combination of back pain with weakness and the presence of urinary disturbance, together with the band-like sensation characteristic of a sensory level. The clinical examination confirmed an upper motor neuron pattern of weakness, and urgent spinal imaging was indicated as treating this condition early may prevent paralysis.

KEY POINTS

- Suspected spinal cord compression is a neurological emergency and requires urgent diagnosis and treatment
- Bladder disturbance, leg weakness and the sensory level are 'red flag' symptoms and signs that should raise alarm
- Early treatment of spinal cord compression with steroids or surgery may prevent paralysis

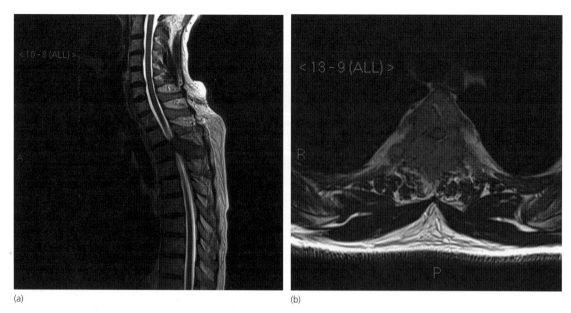

(a)   (b)

Figure 2.2 MRI showing malignant cord compression in the thoracic spine.

Further reading and references

Abrahm JL, Banffy MB, Harris MB. Spinal cord compression in
   patients with advanced metastatic cancer: 'all I care about is
   walking and living my life'. *JAMA* 2008;**299**(8):937–46.

A 25-year-old woman with weakness and tingling in her arms and legs

Leanne, a 25-year-old bartender, comes to the hospital with difficulty walking. She is normally fit and well, but a fortnight ago was off work with a stomach upset. Over the past week, she has been experiencing pins and needles in her hands and feet, and over the past few days has been losing the strength in her arms and legs. Yesterday she was unable to reach up to the highest shelves to bring down the pint glasses, and today she is having difficulty walking even a few steps.

What are the key features of the history?

1 How long was the time course of onset?

2 In what order were her limbs affected?

3 Were there sensory symptoms or motor weakness or both? What was the exact distribution?

4 Were there any associated symptoms?
- Speech or swallowing disturbance
- Diplopia
- Breathlessness
- Urinary retention
- Constipation

5 What was the preceding illness; was there any diarrhoea or a respiratory tract infection?

Her symptoms came on over the 7 days prior to admission. Initially she noticed numbness on the soles of both feet, which gradually spread up to her knees, and over the course of a few days reached her hands. At that time she also had difficulty getting up from the chair, and now her arms are weak as well. She has not had any double vision, but on one or two occasions, when she was swallowing liquids, she complained that they would go up her nose and she would choke. She was not breathless. Bowel and bladder functions

Neurology: Clinical Cases Uncovered, 1st edition. © M. Macleod, M. Simpson and S. Pal. Published 2011 by Blackwell Publishing Ltd.

were normal, but, 2 weeks prior to the symptoms, she had had a 3-day bout of profuse diarrhoea.

What is the likely differential diagnosis?

Leanne describes a combination of sensory and motor symptoms, affecting all four limbs. This could be compatible with a lesion either in the cervical spinal cord (above the level which supplies the arms) or with a peripheral nerve disorder. However, the associated swallowing difficulties would not be produced by a lesion in the spinal cord, and the order of progression of symptoms (feet first, followed by knees, followed by hands) would be in keeping with a length-dependent peripheral neuropathy.

If the patient complained of a 'band-like sensation' around the trunk, this would suggest a sensory level, and would argue strongly in favour of spinal cord disease. Similarly, urinary retention and constipation are alarm symptoms of spinal cord compression, and are much less common with peripheral neuropathies, although they can sometimes occur because of associated autonomic neuropathy. Peripheral neuropathies can also affect bulbar function (causing dysarthria and dysphagia), respiratory muscle function (causing type 2 respiratory failure) or eye movements (causing diplopia and ophthalmoplegia). Preceding gastrointestinal symptoms suggest a post-infectious aetiology.

What are the key features of the examination?

Overall, the history is most suggestive of a length-dependent peripheral neuropathy and the examination should be targeted towards confirming this. The main purpose of the examination is to distinguish a spinal cord lesion (upper motor neuron) from a peripheral nerve disorder (lower motor neuron). It is also necessary to look for any complications of these conditions, such as unstable blood pressure, tachycardia (autonomic neuropathy) or respiratory failure (peripheral neuropathy), or urinary retention (spinal cord disease).

On examination, the pulse and blood pressure were normal. Eye movements were full and there was no diplopia. She had slight difficulty swallowing water, but the voice was normal, the cough was good and there was no facial weakness. The cranial nerves were otherwise normal. The limbs were normal on inspection, with no wasting or fasciculations. Tone was reduced, power was reduced symmetrically to 3/5 in all muscle groups in the legs and 4/5 throughout the arms. Sensation was altered in all modalities in the legs to knee level and in the arms to mid-forearm level, in a glove and stocking pattern. There was no sensory level. All of the reflexes were absent and the plantars were mute.

> ### Box 3.1 Spirometry
>
> Respiratory muscle strength can be assessed by measuring vital capacity, using a spirometer. This is not the same as peak expiratory flow rate. Peak flow meters are more widely available than vital capacity spirometers; however they only determine whether there is bronchoconstriction and *do not* accurately test respiratory muscle function. Therefore, the peak flow rate may be misleading as it is possible to have a normal peak flow rate in the presence of significant respiratory muscle weakness.

The examination findings are in keeping with a lower motor neuron problem. The history is relatively short, hence there is no evidence of muscle wasting or fasciculations (which take longer to develop). There is no evidence of autonomic nervous system involvement. There is nothing in the examination to suggest spinal cord disease. The likely diagnosis is Guillain–Barré syndrome, also known as acute inflammatory demyelinating polyradiculoneuropathy. The short history contrasts with chronic inflammatory demyelinating polyneuropathy; in the former, the illness reaches a peak within 4 weeks, while in the latter it would still be progressing at this stage.

What investigations are required?

The diagnosis of Guillain–Barré syndrome is made predominantly on the basis of clinical history and examination, but certain tests are useful to monitor for complications, confirm the diagnosis and exclude other conditions.

Vital capacity

Guillain–Barré syndrome can be fatal, and the majority of deaths occur because of respiratory muscle involvement. Therefore, it is *essential* that all patients with suspected or confirmed Guillain–Barré syndrome should have their vital capacity monitored regularly (at least four times per day, or more frequently if worsening). This can be done at the bedside with a vital capacity monitor (Box 3.1). As a guide, readings of <15 ml/kg (i.e. <1.0 L for a 70 kg adult) indicate life-threatening respiratory involvement, and the patient requires urgent intubation and transfer to the intensive care unit. However, it is the trend in readings that is important, rather than the absolute values, and if the vital capacity is falling rather than

remaining stable, the patient should be assessed *early* by the intensive care unit with a view to transfer before the situation becomes critical.

ECG and blood pressure measurement

Guillain–Barré syndrome can involve the autonomic nervous system and can cause cardiac arrhythmias. In the acute stages of the illness, patients should be attached to a cardiac monitor as this is another cause of death in this group. Autonomic involvement can also cause lability of blood pressure, which may require treatment.

Nerve conduction studies

Nerve conduction studies are very useful in confirming the clinical diagnosis of Guillain–Barré syndrome and other neuropathies, and can also provide information about prognosis. They use electrical signals to measure the conduction velocity and amplitude of signals in motor and sensory nerves. The velocity of the fastest conducting nerve fibres is calculated by measuring the distance (in millimetres) between a stimulating electrode at one point on the nerve and a recording electrode at another point, and dividing this by the time (in milliseconds) that it takes a signal to travel between the two points. The reason that nerve signals can travel so fast (normal conduction velocity in the median nerve is >50 m/s) is because they are covered in myelin sheaths which insulate the 'wires' and allow faster transfer of electrical information. In Guillain–Barré syndrome, the central pathological process is *demyelination* of peripheral nerves, thus nerve conduction becomes slower.

Nerve conduction studies can also measure the amplitude of the collective action potentials in a particular nerve. Larger amplitudes reflect a larger number of nerve

Table 3.1 Variants of Guillain–Barré syndrome (GBS).

Disease	Characteristics	Antibody
Acute inflammatory demyelinating polyneuropathy (AIDP)	'Classic' GBS; demyelination on nerve conduction studies (NCS)	Not known
Chronic inflammatory demyelinating polyneuropathy (CIDP)	Slower onset, longer course which may be relapsing and remitting. Demyelination on NCS	Not known
Miller–Fisher syndrome	Ataxia, ophthalmoplegia, areflexia; demyelination (sensory > motor) on NCS	Anti-GQ1b
Acute motor axonal neuropathy (AMAN)	Motor involvement only; axonal damage *without demyelination* on NCS	Anti-ganglioside antibodies (GM1, GD1)
Acute motor and sensory axonal neuropathy (AMSAN)	Motor and sensory involvement; axonal damage on NCS	Anti-ganglioside antibodies (GM1, GD1)
Bickerstaff's encephalitis	Ophthalmoplegia, ataxia, encephalopathy, areflexia	Anti-GQ1b

fibres in the axon conducting the signal. In some forms of Guillain–Barré syndrome, and in other neuropathies, there is damage to the nerve axons as well as (or instead of) the myelin sheaths, causing some nerve fibres to die off and producing an action potential of a smaller amplitude. It is generally easier for nerves to recover from demyelination than it is from axonal damage, hence the forms of Guillain–Barré syndrome with axonal damage tend to be more severe and produce longer lasting disability. The variants of Guillain–Barré syndrome are summarised in Table 3.1.

Lumbar puncture

Examination of cerebrospinal fluid (CSF) in Guillain–Barré syndrome characteristically shows $<5 \times 10^6$ white cells, with an elevated protein and normal glucose ratio. CSF white cell counts of greater than $10 \times 10^6/cm^3$ suggest an alternative diagnosis, such as Lyme disease, viral encephalomyelitis (due to agents such as West Nile virus, poliovirus or enterovirus 71) or human immunodeficiency virus (HIV) infection, where a Guillain–Barré-like illness can occur during seroconversion. HIV should always be considered in the differential diagnosis of Guillain–Barré syndrome, even with a normal CSF white cell count.

Blood tests

• Urea and electrolytes: to exclude hypokalaemia (another cause of acute flaccid tetraparesis)
• Liver function tests: may be deranged in Guillain–Barré syndrome
• Erythrocyte sedimentation rate (ESR): may be elevated
• Creatine kinase: to exclude myopathy as a cause of tetraparesis
• Immunoglobulin levels: need to be measured before starting intravenous immunoglobulin (IVIG), one of the treatments for Guillain–Barré syndrome, as IgA deficiency can cause anaphylactic shock in response to IVIG
• Consider HIV testing
• Consider serology for Lyme disease (*Borrelia burgdoferi*)
• Consider testing antibodies such as anti-ganglioside and anti-GQ1b which are associated with subtypes of Guillain–Barré syndrome (Table 3.1)

Her vital capacity was measured at 3.0L, which was in the normal range for her size. The ECG showed a heart rate of 80 beats per minute, blood pressure was 130/70 mmHg without postural drop, and routine blood tests were normal. Lumbar puncture showed an acellular CSF with an elevated protein level of 1.5 g/L (0.1–0.45 g/L) but normal glucose ratio. Nerve conduction studies showed widespread slowing of conduction in sensory and motor nerves, in keeping with the diagnosis of Guillain–Barré syndrome.

What causes Guillain–Barré syndrome?

The disease is thought to be autoimmune in origin, and two-thirds of cases have a preceding infection, usually a few weeks before the onset of neurological symptoms. These include *Campylobacter jejuni*, cytomegalovirus (CMV), Epstein–Barr virus (EBV) and *Mycoplasma pneumoniae*. The putative mechanism is that there is a structural similarity between the infectious agent and the peripheral nerve (referred to as 'molecular mimicry'), such that the immune system recognises peripheral nerve antigens as pathogens and directs an inappropriate response against them, with anti-ganglioside antibodies. The preceding infectious organism can also influence the clinical course of the disease; for example, antecedent *C. jejuni* infection (which is particularly common in northern China) is associated with axonal rather than demyelinating nerve damage and antecedent EBV infection is usually associated with a milder course of Guillain–Barré syndrome. By the time Guillain–Barré syndrome develops, there is no benefit in treating the infection with antibiotics or antivirals.

How should a patient with Guillain–Barré syndrome be managed?

Monitoring and supportive treatment

Regular measurement of vital capacity and early discussion with intensive care in the event of deteriorating or unsatisfactory readings is essential. Cardiac monitoring is indicated in the acute phase of the illness and should be continued until the patient begins to recover. Patients also need prophylaxis against deep vein thrombosis and treatment for constipation as they are at high risk of these complications of immobility.

Disease-modifying treatment

As Guillain–Barré syndrome is a disease of autoimmune aetiology, treatment is given with the aim of modulating the immune system. IVIG is generally used as first-line therapy, and is given via a peripheral intravenous cannula as a slow infusion over several hours for five consecutive days (Box 3.2). The dose used in Guillain–Barré syndrome is 0.4 g/kg/day. The evidence in favour of IVIG was obtained from trials in non-ambulant patients with symptoms lasting less than 2 weeks prior to initiation of

> ### Box 3.2 Intravenous immunoglobulin (IVIG)
>
> - Intravenous immunoglobulin is prepared from the pooled plasma of around 8000 blood donors. It consists largely of IgG, with small amounts of IgA and IgM
> - It was first used in the treatment of thrombotic thrombocytopenic purpura, and has since been used in a variety of autoimmune diseases, although its mechanism of action is unknown
> - Common side effects include headache, myalgia, flushing and fever. Rare but serious risks of IVIG include acute renal failure (particularly in patients with pre-existing renal impairment; this can be reduced by adequate pre-hydration), anaphylaxis (particularly in patients with IgA deficiency; this risk can be reduced by using an IgA-free preparation) and the theoretical risks of transmission of infectious agents associated with all blood products
> - Some patients may have ethical or religious objections to treatment with blood products

treatment; IVIG should therefore be given as early as possible, and the evidence for its use later on in the illness or in patients with milder disease, who are still ambulant, is less clear. In this circumstance, plasma exchange may be more appropriate.

The alternative to IVIG is plasma exchange, which involves venesection of large amounts of blood, which is then circulated through a cell separator machine. In this way, the plasma (which contains the antibodies thought to be responsible for the nerve damage in Guillain–Barré syndrome) is filtered and a plasma substitute is returned to the body via another vein. The process is time-consuming and more invasive than IVIG, although it is equally effective, and is used for patients in whom IVIG is ineffective or contraindicated. There is no place for steroids in the management of Guillain–Barré syndrome.

Symptomatic treatment

Patients may complain of pain or paraesthesiae, often localised to the lower back or legs, and this can be ameliorated by simple analgesics (paracetamol, ibuprofen) or agents used in the treatment of neuropathic pain (gabapentin or carbamazepine).

Leanne was started on a 5-day course of intravenous immunoglobulin and her weakness progressed no further. Her vital capacity was monitored regularly and remained stable. She was troubled by feelings of pins-and-needles in all four limbs, which kept her awake at night. She began intensive physiotherapy and was able to walk a few steps. She wondered whether she would be left like this for ever.

What is the likely outcome?

Even with currently available immunotherapy and intensive care, Guillain–Barré syndrome still carries an appreciable mortality of around 5%. Deaths are largely due to unrecognised respiratory muscle involvement (up to 25% of patients have respiratory involvement sufficiently severe to require mechanical ventilation), cardiac arrhythmias or the complications of immobility. Eighty per cent of patients recover fully with no persisting disability. A poorer outcome is more likely in males, older patients or where there is neurophysiological evidence of axonal damage or preceding CMV infection. However, even in those who recover completely, this can take a long time – recovery may continue for up to 2 years – and patients may require prolonged inpatient rehabilitation.

By definition, Guillain–Barré syndrome reaches its maximal severity within 4 weeks of onset, although more commonly within 2 weeks. It is generally monophasic, and relapses are rare. The related illness, chronic inflammatory demyelinating polyradiculoneuropathy (CIDP) is similar to Guillain–Barré, but the onset is more insidious, over several weeks to months, and the disease can follow a relapsing and remitting course (Box 3.2). Patients with CIDP can require multiple courses of IVIG, and there *is* a role for high-dose oral steroids in this condition. Other treatments that have been used include azathioprine, methotrexate and cyclosporin, although there is no randomised controlled trial evidence to support their efficacy.

CASE REVIEW

This patient presents with a classic history of Guillain–Barré syndrome, with subacute onset of weakness and altered sensation in all four limbs, with a preceding diarrhoeal illness. She was carefully monitored for respiratory failure and autonomic instability, and was treated with intravenous immunoglobulin with a good outcome. Patients with Guillain–Barré syndrome may be very unwell and deteriorate rapidly, and their treating doctors must have a low threshold for involving the intensive care unit; although it is a treatable condition, it still has a significant mortality.

KEY POINTS

- Guillain–Barré syndrome causes a length-dependent demyelinating peripheral neuropathy, believed to be of autoimmune origin
- Patients with Guillain–Barré syndrome may become very unwell and die from autonomic involvement, pulmonary embolism or respiratory failure. They therefore require close monitoring and prompt identification and treatment of any deterioration
- Guillain–Barré syndrome is treated with intravenous immunoglobulin or plasma exchange; these are equivalent in terms of efficacy but immunoglobulin is more readily available and less invasive

Further reading and references

van Doorn PA, Ruts L, Jacobs BC. Clinical features, pathogenesis, and treatment of Guillain–Barré syndrome. *Lancet Neurol* 2008:**7**(10);939–50.

PART 2: CASES

Case 4 A 45-year-old man with uncontrollable seizures

Keith is a 45-year-old nurse who was driving home after a night shift when he noticed his fuel light was flashing. He pulled over to the petrol station but while he was filling up the tank, collapsed to the ground, became stiff and started shaking. The service station attendant, who was a first-aider, rushed out to find him and realised he was having a seizure. As he had learned on the first aid course, he noted the time on his watch (9.15 am) and called an ambulance. By the time the ambulance driver arrived, the man was still fitting, and the paramedics drove him to the emergency department with the sirens blaring. They arrived at hospital at 9.55 am, and the seizure showed no sign of stopping.

What is the diagnosis?

The patient fulfils the diagnostic criteria for status epilepticus, a condition where there is continuous epileptic activity for 30 minutes or more, or where there are multiple seizures without recovery of consciousness in between. Like all epileptic seizures, status epilepticus can be generalised (as in this patient) or partial (also called non-convulsive status). Non-convulsive status may be harder to recognise, and can go unnoticed, particularly in patients with intellectual disability or other underlying brain disease.

Who gets status epilepticus?

In children, status epilepticus occurs most commonly in association with intellectual disability or a structural brain lesion, particularly in the frontal lobes. In adults, it most often occurs as the first presentation of epilepsy, usually due to other cerebral pathology such as encephalitis, stroke, brain tumour or metabolic upset. It can also occur in patients with established epilepsy.

Non-convulsive status epilepticus is almost certainly under-diagnosed in patients with learning disability. In patients with known epilepsy or structural brain disease who present with non-specific drowsiness or global neurological deterioration, an electroencephalograph (EEG) may be extremely useful in diagnosing non-convulsive seizure activity which is otherwise not clinically apparent.

How should Keith's status epilepticus be managed?

Status epilepticus has a high mortality of 10–20% and, with increasing durations of seizures, there is a high risk of neuronal damage, which may be permanent. It is a medical emergency. A summary of the management is shown in Box 4.1.

In patients without known epilepsy, and where there is no obvious metabolic cause for the status epilepticus, urgent brain imaging with CT or MRI is mandatory to exclude a structural lesion. In patients who are febrile or who have a headache, lumbar puncture (LP) should be considered to rule out encephalitis.

The patient arrived in A&E and was taken straight to the resuscitation room. He was tachycardic, febrile at 38°C and hypotensive at 100/60 mmHg. He was given oxygen, cannulated, and given two doses of lorazepam 4 mg i.v. with no effect on his seizures. He had no history of seizures and was not taking any medicines, so he was loaded with phenytoin 15 mg/kg i.v. After 30 minutes, he was still fitting, and the emergency registrar fast-paged the intensive care unit (ICU). He was intubated, paralysed and ventilated, and an urgent EEG was recorded. The EEG showed that he was no longer having seizures and he was monitored on the ICU. He was taken for a CT scan of the brain, which was normal with no evidence of stroke or structural lesion to account for his status epilepticus.

The Intensive Care House Officer called the patient's wife to find out if he had ever had seizures before. She

Neurology: Clinical Cases Uncovered, 1st edition. © M. Macleod, M. Simpson and S. Pal. Published 2011 by Blackwell Publishing Ltd.

> **Box 4.1 Emergency management of convulsive (generalised) status epilepticus**
>
> **Resuscitation**
> - Airway
> - Breathing
> - Circulation
> - i.v. access
> - Oxygen
>
> **Investigation**
> - Glucose (and treat hypoglycaemia promptly)
> - Bloods for electrolytes, calcium, magnesium, full blood count, clotting
> - Where appropriate, antiepileptic drug levels, alcohol level, toxicology screen
> - Consider need for brain imaging/lumbar puncture (once patient is resuscitated)
>
> **Therapy**
> - Benzodiazepines (e.g. diazepam, lorazepam, midazolam), which can be administered intravenously, buccally or rectally depending on routes available. NB pay attention to need for airway maintenance with increasing doses
> - Phenytoin (loading dose given intravenously, in adults 15 mg/kg in normal saline over 30–60 minutes) – lower dose if patient is already on phenytoin
> - Call ICU early – other potential treatments include intravenous phenobarbitone and propofol, which should only be given with anaesthetic facilities available

said no, but she had been worried about him because he had been behaving oddly for the past couple of days and complaining of headache, and had been aggressive towards their cat the previous evening. He was normally a very kind and gentle man, and never smoked or drank alcohol, although she thought he was behaving like a drunk. The ICU doctors performed a lumbar puncture, which showed 200 lymphocytes (normal range <5), 2 red cells and a protein of 0.98 (normal range <0.45 g/L). He was treated for viral encephalitis and 2 days later the polymerase chain reaction (PCR) test for herpes simplex virus (HSV) came back positive.

In this patient a clear cause has been identified for his status epilepticus; the patient has herpex simplex viral encephalitis, which is highly epileptogenic. The history of a subacute change in personality combined with headache and seizures was the clue to this diagnosis, which is confirmed on lumbar puncture. However, if it is suspected, treatment should begin before the investigation results are obtained. Viral encephalitis may also produce structural changes in the brain and patients may therefore be at risk of epilepsy in the longer term, as well as changes to memory and personality and a variety of other neurological deficits.

Keith was extubated, regained consciousness and returned to the ward, where he was making good progress. He continued treatment with intravenous aciclovir and regular phenytoin to control seizures, and was beginning to mobilise around the ward with the aid of the physiotherapist. One week later, however, he seemed drowsy and irritable, and did not want to get out of bed. The House Officer had great difficulty in waking him up, and when she did, he appeared very slow and confused. She ordered an EEG which showed constant epileptic activity (Fig. 4.1). He was in non-convulsive status and was treated aggressively with antiepileptic drugs.

EEGs in status epilepticus

An EEG (Fig. 4.2) is useful for all patients with status epilepticus to assess the control of seizures in patients who are paralysed and ventilated, and to confirm the diagnosis; it is not uncommon for patients with pseudo-seizures, which are characteristically very prolonged, to be intubated in the intensive care unit, being treated unnecessarily with anticonvulsants. Furthermore, an EEG is the only way to definitively diagnose non-convulsive status. Certain causes of status epilepticus (e.g. herpes simplex encephalitis) have characteristic patterns on EEG, with most marked seizure activity over the temporal lobes.

One week later, Keith was once again alert and mobilising. He completed his course of antiviral therapy and was eventually discharged home. He was unable to return to his job because his memory remained impaired, but he moved to a house with a garden and began to grow his own vegetables. Because of concerns over the long-term side effects of phenytoin, 6 months after his presentation he was changed to lamotrigine, and 2 years later remained seizure-free on long-term lamotrigine therapy.

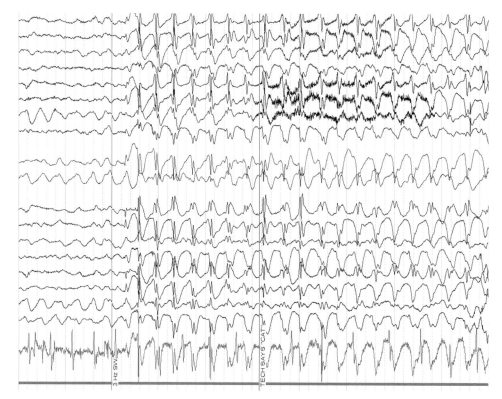

Figure 4.1 EEG of this patient showing the onset of continuous spike-wave epileptic activity.

CASE REVIEW

This patient, who did not have a history of epilepsy, presented with status epilepticus. He did not respond to initial treatment and required early admittance to the ICU. In adults without a known precipitant of status epilepticus, it is important to identify the cause, as this may affect the immediate management, as in this case. Herpes simplex encephalitis may cause a subacute change in personality, headache and seizures, and requires prompt treatment with antiviral drugs, even before the diagnosis is confirmed. In this case the patient had a good outcome; however, untreated the mortality is around 70%, and even with appropriate treatment HSV often causes long-term cognitive impairment, memory difficulties, irreversible brain damage and death in around 30%.

KEY POINTS

- Status epilepticus is a medical emergency with a high mortality
- Status epilepticus is defined as continuous epileptic activity for 30 minutes or more, or multiple seizures without recovery of consciousness in between
- Patients in status epilepticus require airway management and early discussion with the intensive care unit if not improving with benzodiazepines and anticonvulsants
- Non-convulsive status should be considered in patients with epilepsy and non-specific alteration in mental status, and an EEG may be required to rule this out

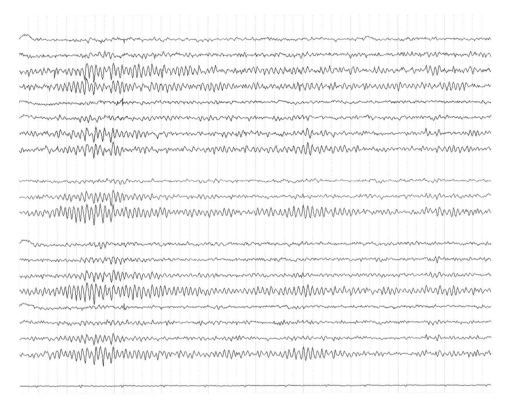

Figure 4.2 A normal EEG.

Further reading and references

Kelso A, Cock H. Status epilepticus. *Pract Neurol* 2005;**5**: 322–33.

Kennedy PG. Viral encephalitis. *J Neurol* 2005;**252**(3):268–72.

Solomon T, Hart IJ, Beeching NJ. Viral encephalitis: a clinician's guide. *Pract Neurol* 2007;**7**(5):288–305.

Case 5 A 24-year-old woman with headaches and abnormal optic fundi

Ashley, a 24-year-old waitress, is referred urgently from her optician. She has been having headaches for a few months and thought she might need glasses. The optician took one look in her fundi and sent her straight to hospital.

What are the key features of the history?

The majority of headaches can be diagnosed on the basis of the history, therefore it is essential to have a careful and methodical approach. The neurologist must be able to distinguish *secondary headaches* (headaches as a result of underlying brain pathology) from *primary headaches* (headaches without underlying brain pathology); this is discussed further in Cases 20 and 25.

1 What is the duration of the headaches and how often does she get them?
2 What is the location and character of the headaches?
   • Unilateral or bilateral
   • Throbbing, dull, aching or sharp
3 Are there any factors that make the headaches worse?
   • Coughing, bending, sneezing
   • Lying down
   • Eye movement
4 Are there any associated symptoms?
   • Nausea, vomiting
   • Visual obscurations
   • Visual blurring, double vision, visual loss
   • Tinnitus, hearing loss
   • Photophobia
   • Seizures
   • Personality change
   • Limb weakness or altered sensation
5 Are there any systemic symptoms, particularly alarm symptoms that might suggest a malignancy?
6 Has she commenced any new medications recently?

Neurology: Clinical Cases Uncovered, 1st edition. © M. Macleod, M. Simpson and S. Pal. Published 2011 by Blackwell Publishing Ltd.

She first developed the headaches about 3 months ago, and they have got gradually worse over this time; prior to this she has never had headaches. They are present daily, localised to the front of her head behind the eyes, and are worst in the morning. By the time she has got up and got into the shower, they are a good deal better. She feels nauseous with the headache, and has vomited on one or two occasions. She notices that the headache is worse while she is bending over and retching. She has also been having some trouble with her vision. At times, she notices 'bits missing' from her visual field, mainly in the centre, and this lasts for only a few seconds. At times she notices double vision, particularly when looking to the side. In general she has been otherwise well, although 6 months ago she broke her ankle playing volleyball, and since then she has gained around 12.5 kg in weight. She takes no regular medications.

!RED FLAG

There are a number of features about this history which should ring alarm bells for *raised intracranial pressure*:

   • Worst in the morning, improving over the day
   • Worse on bending or retching
   • Associated with nausea and vomiting (this can also occur with migraine)
   • Visual obscurations
   • Double vision

What are the key features of the examination?

In patients with suspected raised intracranial pressure (ICP), the examination should include the following:

1 Conscious level.
2 Pulse and blood pressure (raised ICP can cause hypertension and bradycardia via the Cushing response) (Box 5.1).

> ### Box 5.1 Physiology of raised intracranial pressure
>
> - The skull is a closed box (Monroe–Kellie doctrine)
> - Therefore, any increase in its contents (e.g. from cerebral haemorrhage or tumour) must be compensated for by a physiological decrease in blood flow or CSF volume
> - If the increase in skull contents is too great to be compensated for in this way, intracranial pressure increases
> - This is linked to systemic blood pressure by the following equation:
>
>   Cerebral perfusion pressure = mean arterial blood pressure − intracranial pressure
>
> - Therefore, when intracranial pressure rises, cerebral perfusion pressure falls, and the brain is liable to ischaemic injury

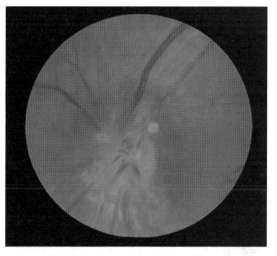

Figure 5.1 Papilloedema.

A right 6th nerve palsy – "look right", patient reports horizontal diplopia on right lateral gaze

Figure 5.2 Sixth nerve palsy.

3 General examination for features of a primary malignancy.

4 Visual field examination looking for peripheral field defects, which might localise an intracerebral lesion, or enlargement of the blind spot which can occur due to pressure on the optic nerve in raised ICP.

5 Eye movements looking for 6th (and rarely 3rd) nerve palsies, which can be 'false localising signs' reflecting raised ICP (both nerves run a long intracranial course and are liable to compression along the way).

6 Fundoscopy looking for papilloedema or loss of spontaneous retinal vein pulsation, another feature of raised ICP (Fig. 5.1).

7 Document visual acuities and colour vision (papilloedema may eventually become sight-threatening).

8 General neurological examination looking for focal signs that might localise a brain lesion further.

Ashley is obese with a body mass index of 32. Her heart rate is 70 beats/min and her blood pressure is 130/90 mmHg. She is fully alert and orientated. On examination of the cranial nerves, she has horizontal diplopia on lateral gaze bilaterally with incomplete abduction of both eyes. She has normal peripheral fields but enlarged blind spots in both eyes, and bilateral papilloedema with loss of spontaneous retinal vein pulsation. There are no other abnormalities on examination of the cranial nerves or the limbs.

What is the differential diagnosis now?

The examination shows evidence of bilateral 6th nerve palsies, enlarged blind spots and bilateral papilloedema (Fig. 5.2); like the history, these findings are suggestive of raised intracranial pressure. However, there are no signs or symptoms that suggest a focal lesion, such as limb weakness, sensory loss or ataxia, and there is no history of seizures (which are relatively common with brain lesions). There are no systemic symptoms that would point towards an underlying malignancy.

Raised ICP may be primary (called idiopathic intracranial hypertension), or secondary to a variety of causes, such as brain tumour, cerebral haematoma, venous sinus thrombosis, hydrocephalus or meningitis. In any case, the patient requires urgent imaging to exclude a space-occupying lesion. Ideally this should be an MRI scan with magnetic resonance venography (MRV) to examine the cerebral venous sinuses, although if this will result in delay a CT scan with contrast should be performed instead. If these are normal, a lumbar puncture should be performed to exclude meningitis and to measure the CSF pressure (Box 5.2).

PART 2: CASES

Box 5.2 Lumbar puncture and headache

If there is a history suggestive of raised intracranial pressure, brain imaging is mandatory before lumbar puncture. If a lumbar puncture is performed in someone who has a brain tumour or other space-occupying lesion, there is a risk that removal of CSF may lead to 'coning' – downwards displacement of the brain through the tentorium and foramen magnum, with compression of vital structures and ultimately coma and death.

The CT brain scan with contrast is normal. An MRI scan with MRV is also normal. There is no space-occupying lesion and no venous sinus thrombosis. A lumbar puncture is performed which shows an opening pressure of 35 cmH₂O (normal range 8–20 cmH₂O), a white cell count of 0, red cell count of 5, normal protein and glucose. Following the lumbar puncture, she reports that her headache feels better.

These results have excluded secondary causes of raised ICP, and confirm the likely diagnosis of idiopathic intracranial hypertension (IIH).

What causes idiopathic intracranial hypertension?

The cause is not known. One theory is that there is an obstruction to CSF outflow, either at the level of the arachnoid villi or the dural venous sinuses (although any obstructing clots in this area are too small to be seen on standard brain imaging).

How should idiopathic intracranial hypertension be managed?

IIH was previously known as 'benign' intracranial hypertension, because it was not caused by a brain tumour (i.e. it was non-malignant). However, this often led to a degree of complacency in management, sometimes resulting in irreversible visual failure. There are several potential management strategies, although there is no high-quality evidence base to support them. They include:

1 Lifestyle modifications: weight loss.
2 Symptomatic treatments: analgesia, anti-emetics.
3 Diuretics: acetazolamide, thiazides, loop diuretics.
4 Lumbar puncture (repeated if necessary).
5 Surgical procedures: lumboperitoneal shunt, ventriculoperitoneal shunt, optic nerve sheath fenestration (potential complications of shunts include shunt block-

age and infection, low pressure headache and subdural haemorrhage; potential complications of optic nerve sheath fenestration include visual loss, orbital haemorrhage and glaucoma).

Ashley is commenced on acetazolamide and an appointment is made with the dietician. She found the lumbar puncture so unpleasant that she will do anything to avoid another one. She joins a running club and manages to lose 12.5 kg in weight. Her headaches improve and her vision remains normal. After 6 months she is able to stop the diuretics.

CASE REVIEW

This patient presents with signs and symptoms of raised intracranial pressure, which should raise alarm bells and requires urgent investigation. Brain imaging with CT and MRI/MRV exclude a structural lesion and a lumbar puncture shows normal constituents but a raised opening pressure, consistent with idiopathic intracranial hypertension. Sometimes this condition requires urgent surgical treatment (if there is evidence of visual loss), but most patients can be managed with lumbar puncture, diuretics and lifestyle modifications.

KEY POINTS

- Symptoms of raised intracranial pressure include morning headache with vomiting, worsening with coughing or bending, and visual symptoms of diplopia or obscurations
- Signs of raised intracranial pressure include papilloedema, enlarged blind spot, 6th nerve palsy, 3rd nerve palsy and sometimes visual loss (late)
- These symptoms and signs should raise alarm bells and require urgent brain imaging
- When secondary causes have been excluded, a lumbar puncture may be necessary to confirm the diagnosis of idiopathic intracranial hypertension

Further reading and references

Binder DK, Horton JC, Lawton MT, McDermott MW. Idiopathic intracranial hypertension. *Neurosurgery* 2004;**54**(3):538–51.

Skau M, Brennum J, Gjerris F, Jensen R. What is new about idiopathic intracranial hypertension? An updated review of mechanism and treatment. *Cephalalgia* 2006;**26**(4):384–99.

Case 6   A 37-year-old man with sudden, severe headache

A 37-year-old man experienced the sudden onset of a severe headache while playing squash one lunchtime. The headache reached a maximum intensity instantly. He felt sore and stiff all the way up the back of his neck, didn't like bright lights, felt sick and within 15 minutes he started vomiting.

What are the key features of the history?

1 How long did it take the headache to reach its maximum severity?
- Instantaneous or gradual
- Length of time it built over

2 How long did the headache last for?

3 What other symptoms did he have?
- Nausea
- Vomiting
- Photophobia, phonophobia
- Loss of consciousness
- Visual disturbance
- Speech disturbance
- Motor or sensory symptoms

4 What is his past medical history?
- Past history of migraine
- Vascular disease elsewhere
- Vascular risk factors: smoking, hypertension
- Alcohol misuse

5 Is there a family history of similar problems?
- Migraine
- Aneurysms
- Intracranial haemorrhage/sudden death

The history is the *most essential* part of the assessment of patients with sudden, severe headache because it helps

Neurology: Clinical Cases Uncovered, 1st edition. © M. Macleod, M. Simpson and S. Pal. Published 2011 by Blackwell Publishing Ltd.

refine your differential diagnosis. The majority (40%) of people presenting to hospital with sudden severe headache will have a benign thunderclap headache, only about one in four will have suffered a subarachnoid haemorrhage (SAH).

SAH usually presents with a characteristic combination of symptoms (Box 6.1). Headache and meningism are due to irritation of the meninges by subarachnoid blood. Loss of consciousness or sudden death may be due to a sharp rise in intracranial pressure with consequent reduced cerebral perfusion. Focal neurological symptoms are uncommon, and may relate to focal ischaemia due to vessel spasm or to mass effect from any associated intracerebral haemorrhage.

Almost all conscious patients with SAH complain of headache – in one-third it is the only symptom (Fig. 6.1). The speed with which the headache reaches its maximal intensity is a very important part of the history; in SAH it is rapid – half of those with SAH describe it as instantaneous ('like being hit over the head with a cricket bat'), a further fifth say it develops over 1–5 minutes, and the rest find it escalates over >5 minutes. However, the speed of onset cannot be relied on to identify all cases of SAH, and some present with a more gradual onset. Similarly, while the headache usually persists for several days it may last for only a couple of hours.

Your patient had the 'worst headache of his life', which reached 10 out of 10 on the pain scale instantly. His squash partner said that he had collapsed and lost consciousness for only a few seconds. At the time of assessment 2 hours later he was confused and remained in pain, with nausea and vomiting.

What is the differential diagnosis now?

The speed and duration of his headache is consistent with subarachnoid haemorrhage. This is an important diagnosis to make, for two reasons. Firstly, the risk of

Box 6.1 Key presentations of subarachnoid haemorrhage

- Sudden, severe headache (maximal immediately or within minutes, and lasting ≥1 hour (usually days))
- Other symptoms of meningism (nausea, vomiting, photophobia and neck stiffness)
- Loss of consciousness
- Epileptic seizure(s)
- Focal neurological symptoms (dysphasia, hemisensory/ motor symptoms)
- Sudden death

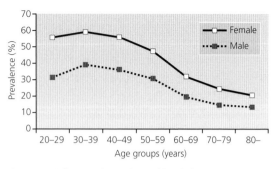

Figure 6.1 Self-reported prevalence of headache.

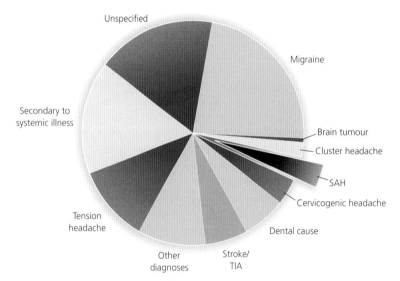

Figure 6.2 Final diagnosis in headache patients assessed in A&E. SAH, subarachnoid haemorrhage; TIA, transient ischaemic attack.

rebleeding for a ruptured aneurysm is high and can be moderated using surgical or endovascular measures. Secondly, there is a risk of vasospasm in the cerebral circulation, which can cause a delayed ischaemic neurological deficit, and this risk can be moderated pharmacologically. It is therefore crucial to establish the cause of headache in this case, and to develop an appropriate management strategy (Box 6.2).

The other symptoms of SAH (Box 6.1) may accompany other causes of sudden severe headache (Fig. 6.2), so they cannot reliably distinguish SAH from the rest. Note that when sudden severe headache is the *only* symptom, one in 10 turn out to have SAH, so the absence of other symptoms cannot be used to 'rule out' SAH. Migraine is unlikely because his symptoms did not evolve and migraine rarely causes loss of consciousness.

Box 6.2 Common causes of sudden, severe headache

- Spontaneous (non-traumatic) subarachnoid haemorrhage
- Headache alone:
  migraine
  cluster headache
  headache associated with sexual activity/exertion
- Headache and other symptoms:
  Vascular (ischaemic and haemorrhagic stroke, arterial dissection)
  infection (meningitis/encephalitis)
  acute hydrocephalus
  intracranial tumour
  intracranial hypotension (spontaneous or following dural puncture)
  metabolic (e.g. phaeochromocytoma)

He had smoked since the age of 15, drank half a bottle of wine per night, and had a sister who had died suddenly of a 'brain haemorrhage' at the age of 27.

What are the key features of the examination?

1 Initial assessment and level of consciousness:
- Airway
- Breathing
- Circulation
- Glasgow Coma Scale (GCS; see p. 74)

2 Evidence for intraparenchymal haemorrhage, vasospasm or complications of raised intracranial pressure:
- Pupillary reaction to light
- Brainstem reflexes
- Visual field defect
- Limb weakness
- Sensory disturbance

3 Systemic examination looking for complications of SAH:
- Blood pressure
- Pulse
- Pulmonary oedema (Box 6.3)
- Fundoscopy

His GCS is 14 (eyes open to voice), his neck is stiff, there are no neurological deficits, and his blood pressure is 180/102 mmHg.

SAH remains the most likely diagnosis. Because SAH is a serious event with a high risk of recurrence and with treatable complications, we need to make substantial efforts to reach a positive diagnosis either of SAH or of an alternative headache syndrome.

> ### Box 6.3 Neurogenic pulmonary oedema (NPO)
>
> - Usually occurs within 4 hours of subarachnoid haemorrhage
> - One-third present with pink frothy sputum
> - 90% of patients with NPO have bilateral diffuse infiltrates on chest X-ray
> - Majority of patients recover within 3 days, but 10% die
> - Management:
>   oxygen support
>   vasoactive drugs

What investigations are required?

1 Full blood count.
2 Urea and electrolytes.
3 Serum glucose.
4 Chest X-ray.
5 12-lead electrocardiogram.
6 Unenhanced CT brain: the investigation of choice for SAH is unenhanced computed tomography (CT) of the brain, performed as soon as possible after headache onset. CT of the brain should be done immediately if consciousness is impaired. Any delay in CT scanning allows subarachnoid blood time to degrade and increases the possibility of a normal scan; ~7% of SAH cannot be seen on CT after 24 hours, and subarachnoid blood is almost completely reabsorbed within 10 days. Subarachnoid blood appears as increased signal intensity on an unenhanced CT scan (Fig. 6.3).
7 Lumbar puncture:
- Anyone with suspected SAH and normal brain CT requires a lumbar puncture, following discussion with a specialist at a neuroscience unit. In SAH red blood cells are found in the subarachnoid space – which is what is tapped in a lumbar puncture.
- Most patients with SAH will have a red cell count of 500 or more. However, similar values may also be caused by bleeding into the CSF caused by the lumbar puncture itself. Unless there is any suspicion of an alternative diagnosis such as meningitis, delay lumbar

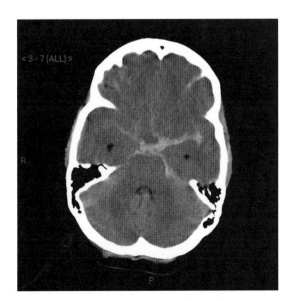

Figure 6.3 CT of the brain in subarachnoid haemorrhage.

puncture for at least 6 hours – preferably 12 hours – after headache onset.

• This is sufficient time to allow haemoglobin from SAH to degrade into both oxyhaemoglobin and bilirubin. Bilirubin signifies SAH because it is only synthesised *in vivo*. In contrast, oxyhaemoglobin – which is often reported in results of CSF spectrophotometry – may form from local bleeding into the CSF at the time of lumbar puncture. The presence of oxyhaemoglobin without bilirubin does not therefore indicate SAH. Oxyhaemoglobin formation is encouraged by physical agitation and increases over time; this is important, because it is not always possible reliably to distinguish between bilirubin and oxyhaemoglobin at spectrophotometry.

• Where patients are scanned soon after headache onset the CT is rarely negative. As time passes not only do the CT changes resolve but the red blood cells within the CSF degrade. When more than a few days have elapsed, the CSF red cell count may be normal; however, bilirubin may remain detectable for up to 3 weeks after SAH, and may be accompanied by elevations in CSF protein and white cell count.

• At lumbar puncture, record or test:
  • CSF opening pressure
  • protein
  • red and white cell counts
  • glucose (compare with serum sample taken at same time)

To minimise any confusion arising from the *in vitro* production of oxyhaemoglobin, the last (i.e. least bloodstained) sample of CSF should be transported to the laboratory by hand and centrifuged immediately. Whether xanthochromia is visible or not, spectrophotometry is necessary to detect bilirubin. The estimation of red cell counts in three consecutive samples of CSF does not reliably distinguish SAH from a traumatic tap.

> *The patient underwent CT scanning, which showed blood in the anterior interhemispheric fissure, confirming the diagnosis of SAH. Other investigations were normal, except an ECG which showed ST-segment elevation and T-wave inversion suggesting myocardial ischaemia.*

The ECG changes are recognisable in SAH; in addition, impaired left ventricular function seen at echocardiography and elevated serum troponin 1 levels are each seen in around 20% of patients, probably due to increased cardiac work due to hypertension and increased circulat-

Box 6.4 ECG changes in subarachnoid haemorrhage	
Normal ECG	38.5%
ST/T changes	46.4%
QTc prolongation	30.6%
Bradycardia	11.7%
Ventricular ectopics	5.7%
2nd/3rd degree AV block	1.6%

ing catecholamines. Each of these are more likely in patients with severe neurological impairment (Box 6.4).

The further investigation of SAH is determined by its likely cause. In some cases SAH occurs in the context of a head injury, and may be accompanied by extradural or subdural haematomas or by diffuse axonal injury (see Case 14). While such cases usually require no further investigation, it is important to rule out the possibility that the head injury might have been the result of a collapse or loss of consciousness caused by SAH rather than vice versa.

Three-quarters of spontaneous SAH are caused by rupture of an intracranial aneurysm, usually of the circle of Willis or its major branches; 20% have no identifiable cause, and at least half of these are probably due to bleeding from veins around the brainstem (perimesencephalic SAH). The remainder are caused by a variety of rare disorders (such as arteriovenous malformations of the brain or spine, arterial dissection, sympathomimetic drugs, tumours and vasculitis).

Multislice CT angiography is the preferred investigation of the underlying cause of spontaneous SAH, because of its speed, tolerability, convenience and the ability to provide 3D reconstructions. CT angiography has a sensitivity and specificity for identifying aneurysms of >90% when compared to the reference standard, catheter angiography (Box 6.5).

> *In this case, CT angiography showed an anterior communicating artery aneurysm consistent with the distribution of blood seen on the CT scan (Fig. 6.4).*

How should patients with SAH be managed?

Management of aneurysmal SAH has three main objectives: to minimise the risk of further bleeding, to prevent and where necessary treat complications, and to promote maximal recovery and return to normal function.

Box 6.5 Sensitivity and specificity of diagnostic tests

- A sensitive test, if negative, is good for ruling out a diagnosis ('snout')
- A specific test, if positive, helps confirm a diagnosis ('spin')
- Where prevalence of aneurysms is 60%, a comparison of CT angiography (CTA) with digital subtraction angiography (DSA) shows:

	DSA +ve	DSA −ve
CTA +ve	54%	3%
CTA −ve	6%	37%

- Sensitivity = 54/60 = 90%; specificity = 37/40 = 91%

Box 6.6 Pivotal clinical trial

The ISAT study was a randomised controlled trial comparing 'clipping' with 'coiling' in 2143 patients with subarachnoid haemorrhage. At 1 year, 30.9% of patients allocated to surgery were dead or disabled, compared with 23.5% of patients allocated to endovascular treatment (NNT = 13.5). The endovascular group had a lower incidence of epilepsy (5.8% vs 10.4%) but a higher rate of late rebleeding (0.6% vs 0.2%).

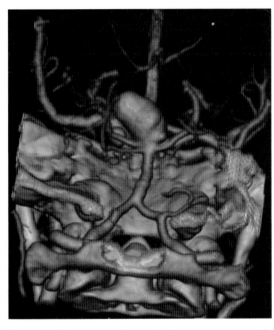

Figure 6.4 CT angiogram of the patient showing an aneurysm of the basilar tip.

Minimising the risk of further bleeding

Following rupture, the risk of rebleeding is substantial – around 25% of patients will have a further bleed within 4 days, and another 25% within the next month. Securing the aneurysm is therefore a matter of priority, and for this reason patients should be transferred, at the earliest opportunity, to a regional neurosciences centre. This is

particularly the case for patients who have no residual problems after their SAH, as they have the most to lose from a further SAH.

Firstly, the anatomy of the aneurysm must be defined to allow a judgement of the feasibility of endovascular ('coiling') or surgical ('clipping') treatment. Where both are feasible and available then endovascular treatment is preferred, as this is associated with reduced death and disability and a reduced incidence of epilepsy at the expense of a slightly increased risk of late rebleeding (Box 6.6).

Endovascular treatment, performed by an interventional neuroradiologist, involves the deployment of fine metal coils within the aneurysm sac through a catheter inserted via the femoral artery. This provides a scaffold on which blood clot can form and has the effect of occluding the aneurysm from the circulation. Risks of the procedure include:

1 Stroke, due to dislodgement of atheroma of, for instance, the aortic arch, dissection of extracranial or intracranial blood vessels, induced vasospasm in intracranial blood vessels, or deployment of coil within the parent vessel rather than the aneurysm.
2 Aneurysm or blood vessel rupture leading to subarachnoid or intracerebral haemorrhage.
3 Local complications in the groin including haemorrhage, infection and femoral nerve palsy.

The continuing exclusion of the aneurysm from the circulation must be confirmed in the months and years ahead with regular check angiography.

Prevention and treatment of complications
Delayed ischaemic neurological deficit
The most important potential complication is vasospasm in the cerebral circulation (Box 6.7). This may lead to

PART 2: CASES

Box 6.7 Risk factors for development of vasospasm

- Thickness of subarachnoid clot on CT
- Early (up to day 5) rise in middle cerebral artery mean flow velocity measured using transcranial Doppler ultrasound
- Glasgow Coma Scale score <14
- Rupture of anterior cerebral or internal carotid artery aneurysm

---

Box 6.8 Pivotal systematic review

A systematic review and meta-analysis of data from three clinical trials involving 783 patients suggests that oral nimodipine reduces the risk of a poor outcome by about 30% (relative risk, 0.70; 95% confidence interval, 0.58–0.84). Two further trials tested nimodipine given first intravenously and then orally, and found no significant benefit (RR, 0.85; 95% CI, 0.57–1.28).

Box 6.9 !Danger – evidence-free zone

Despite vasospasm causing substantial morbidity and mortality, the optimal management of vasospasm following subarachnoid haemorrhage has not been established. Proposed treatments include 'triple H therapy' (hypertension, hydration and hypervolaemia); intra-arterial treatment with vasodilator drugs such as papaverine, magnesium or nimodipine; and angioplasty of the affected vessel. Randomised controlled trials to determine optimal management are urgently required.

---

ischaemia in the brain volume supplied by the affected artery, causing a delayed ischaemic neurological deficit.

Routine treatment with the calcium antagonist nimodipine (60 mg po every 4 hours) has been shown to improve outcome, probably by reducing the incidence of vasospasm, and should be used in all patients unless there is a specific contraindication. The benefits of intravenous nimodipine in patients unable to swallow are not clear (Box 6.8). Other measures that may reduce the incidence of vasospasm include a high fluid intake to avoid hypovolaemia and the avoidance of factors that may induce vasospasm – such as cigarette smoking – particularly during the period of highest risk. There is little evidence to guide the treatment of established vasospasm (Box 6.9).

Hydocephalus

CSF is normally absorbed through the arachnoid granulations into the venous sinuses, but the presence of a substantial amount of blood within the CSF can obstruct these, leading to hydrocephalus, which can in turn cause headache, drowsiness and loss of consciousness. This hydrocephalus is usually self-limiting. Where CT scanning has confirmed the diagnosis and excluded an intracranial mass lesion, CSF can be removed by lumbar puncture. Typically, the opening pressure is recorded with a manometer, and CSF is drained until the pressure falls by one-third. This procedure may be repeated if symptoms return, and only if the hydrocephalus persists should more invasive measures, such as the placement of a ventricular access device for external ventricular drainage, or of a lumbo- or ventriculo-peritoneal shunt, be considered.

Electrolyte balance

Patients with SAH may develop: (1) the syndrome of inappropriate antidiuretic hormone secretion (SIADH), leading to a dilutional hyponatraemia; or (2) a cranial salt-wasting state thought to be due to diabetes insipidus and leading to hypernatraemia. Because hypovolaemia may contribute to vasospasm, SIADH should be managed with large volumes of isotonic ('normal') saline rather than with fluid restriction. Patients with hypernatraemia require aggressive fluid replacement (conventionally with half normal saline/5% dextrose) to prevent hypovolaemia, and DDAVP (deamino-D-arginine vasopressin) to limit renal water loss.

Promotion of recovery and of normal function

Subarachnoid haemorrhage is a major physiological stress, and even patients who make an uncomplicated recovery can expect it to be several months before they are back to 'normal'. They and their families may find it difficult to reconcile the outward appearances of full recovery with their continuing difficulties with everyday life and return to work.

Patients who have experienced ischaemic brain injury may have problems with limb weakness or speech, and may benefit from a period of inpatient neuro-rehabilitation. This is particularly the case for patients with ischaemic injury to the frontal lobes following rupture of, for instance, an anterior communicating artery aneurysm, who may have extensive difficulties with relatively straightforward tasks and with disinhibition despite outward appearances of a full recovery.

Further reading and references

Macrea LM, Tram'er MR, Walder B. Spontaneous subarachnoid hemorrhage and serious cardiopulmonary dysfunction – a systematic review. *Resuscitation* 2005;**65**:139–48.

Mistry N, Mathew L, Parry A. Thunderclap headache. *Pract Neurol* 2009;**9**(5):294–7.

Molyneux AJ, Kerr RS, Yu LM, Clarke M, Sneade M, Yarnold JA, Sandercock P; International Subarachnoid Aneurysm Trial (ISAT) Collaborative Group. International subarachnoid aneurysm trial (ISAT) of neurosurgical clipping versus endovascular coiling in 2143 patients with ruptured intracranial aneurysms: a randomised comparison of effects on survival, dependency, seizures, rebleeding, subgroups, and aneurysm occlusion. *Lancet* 2005;**366**(9488):783–5.

Rinkel GJE, Feigin VL, Algra A, van den Bergh WM, Vermeulen M, van Gijn J. Calcium antagonists for aneurysmal subarachnoid haemorrhage. *Cochrane Database Syst Rev* 2005;Issue 1:CD000277. DOI: 10.1002/14651858.CD000277.pub2.

KEY POINTS

- A first hand eye witness account can be crucial where the patient's ability to recall or recount events is impaired
- Because subarachnoid haemorrhage is a serious condition with a high risk of rebleeding, it is important to be alert to it as a possible diagnosis even if this means many patients with severe migraine undergoing CT and lumbar puncture
- A normal CT brain does not exclude SAH – look carefully in the prepontine cisterns, the occipital horns of the lateral ventricles and in the Sylvian fissures
- While the most informative CSF comes from delayed LP, if the differential diagnosis includes meningitis the LP should be carried out as soon as it is considered safe to do so
- To avoid false positive LPs treat the CSF with care – avoid a traumatic tap if possible (get an experienced doctor to do the LP), get the CSF to the lab by hand and quickly, and have it spun down to separate out any red cells straight away

CASE REVIEW

This 37-year-old man presented with a sudden onset of headache. The speed of onset and the associated nausea and vomiting, neck stiffness and photophobia are typical of subarachnoid haemorrhage. This was confirmed at CT, and CT angiography showed an aneurysm of the anterior communicating artery.

Case 7) A 17-year-old girl who becomes unresponsive after a late night

Heather is a 17-year-old hairdresser who is brought to the emergency room one Sunday morning by ambulance. She was at a birthday party the night before and in the early hours of the morning her mother heard a noise from her room and went in to find her shaking on the floor. She tried to wake her up but she was unresponsive so she phoned an ambulance. By the time she reached hospital she was beginning to wake up but remained confused and disorientated.

What are the key features of the history?

1 When did the patient become unresponsive (or, if the event was unwitnessed, when was she last seen well beforehand)?

2 Were there any warning symptoms before the event?

3 What did she look like during the attack? What was she doing with her eyes, face, arms and legs?

4 Had she bitten her tongue or been incontinent of urine?

5 How long did it take her to recover to normal afterwards?

6 Has she ever had any similar attacks before?

Heather arrived at hospital with the ambulance drivers but was unable to give a history. The emergency department doctor, who was very efficient and was hoping to train as a neurologist, telephoned her home to speak to a witness. Her boyfriend had been in her room at the time and saw the whole event from start to finish, and was able to describe it. She had been well the previous day and had attended a birthday party with him. She had a couple of bottles of beer but had certainly not been drunk, and this amount of alcohol was quite normal for her on a Saturday

night. They came home around midnight, but didn't want to go to bed and sat up in her room watching a zombie movie. She had not complained of feeling unwell during the film and when it was over (around 3 am) got up to get a glass of water before going to bed. It was then that she suddenly fell to the ground, without warning. She became stiff, and then started to shake her arms and legs all together for what seemed like a long time, but may only have been a couple of minutes. He was unable to rouse her during the event. Her eyes seemed to roll back, and her jaw was clenched, but she didn't turn her head in either direction and the colour of her face did not change. He didn't think she had wet herself but she had bitten her tongue.

She was still very drowsy by the time the ambulance came, although during the 20-minute ride to hospital she began to wake up. She had no memory of the event. Clinical examination was normal with no focal neurology.

What is the likely differential diagnosis?

There are a number of potential diagnoses to consider in patients presenting with transient loss of consciousness:

• Seizure
• Vasovagal syncope
• Cardiogenic syncope
• Syncope due to postural hypotension
• Hypoglycaemia
• Psychogenic/non-epileptic attacks

In a young woman of this age, the most likely diagnoses would be seizure or syncope (Table 7.1). The witness history is very detailed and strongly suggests that this event was a seizure.

So does Heather have epilepsy?

This event, as far as we know, is a first seizure. It may be an isolated event (around 5% of the population have a seizure at some point in their life) or it may be part of a tendency to recurrent seizures, which defines

Neurology: Clinical Cases Uncovered, 1st edition. © M. Macleod, M. Simpson and S. Pal. Published 2011 by Blackwell Publishing Ltd.

Table 7.1 Factors helping to distinguish between seizure and syncope.

	Seizure	Syncope
Provoking factors	Sleep deprivation	Prolonged standing
	Alcohol or withdrawal	Emotional factors
	Head injury	Intercurrent illness
	CNS pathology	
	Metabolic derangement	
	Flashing lights	
Face colour	Normal or blue	May go pale
Arms and legs	May stiffen then shake (tonic-clonic seizure)	May twitch
Duration	1–3 minutes	<30 seconds (resolves on lying down)
Tongue biting	Often, often lateral	Seldom
Incontinence	Sometimes	Sometimes
Recovery	30–60 minutes, often confused/sleepy	Few minutes (on lying down)

epilepsy. Therefore it is important to take additional history, to try and establish the likelihood of recurrent events in the future and the impact of the potential diagnosis on her life.

Are there any additional features in the history?

1 Does she have any other types of attack?
  • Absences (5–10 seconds of blank staring, occasionally accompanied by blinking or myoclonic jerks, with no memory of the event afterwards)
  • Myoclonic jerks (uncontrollable jerks of some or all limbs lasting 1–2 seconds, in clear consciousness, often in the morning – these can occur on dropping off to sleep as a normal phenomenon)
  • Complex partial seizures (episodes of altered awareness often with lip smacking or manual automatisms, lasting 1–2 minutes)
2 Is there any family history of seizures or epilepsy?
3 Is she taking any medications that might induce seizures?
4 Were there any other precipitants to the seizure?
5 Does she have any early life risk factors for seizures?
  • Febrile convulsion
  • Head injury
  • Prematurity
  • Previous cerebral infection

6 Particularly in children, is there any history of developmental delay or regression?
7 How will the diagnosis of a seizure affect her life?
  • Driving
  • Occupation
  • Activities/hobbies
  • Pregnancy/contraception

Heather denies any similar events. The very efficient emergency doctor asks her about other types of attacks, in particular blank staring spells, or early morning jerks, but she denies all of these. She thinks her cousin on her mother's side used to have seizures when she was a child, but outgrew them. She is not taking any medications other than the combined oral contraceptive pill. No provoking factors can be identified other than sleep deprivation; there are no early life risk factors and no other neurological symptoms.

She has just got her driver's licence and her parents had recently bought her a car for her 18th birthday. She works as a hairdresser and drives to work in a town 50 km away because there are no buses which go there. Her main hobbies are rock-climbing and swimming. She is not planning to become pregnant.

What investigations are required?

Baseline bloods including urea and electrolytes and glucose should be performed in every patient presenting with seizures because metabolic abnormalities such as hypoglycaemia and hyponatraemia can provoke a seizure. Blood alcohol level may be helpful in determining whether intoxication provoked the seizure.

Policies on brain imaging vary according to local procedure. In acutely unwell patients, a CT scan may be more practical and is almost certainly more accessible, but even a normal CT brain scan does not rule out the possibility of a focal brain lesion underlying the epilepsy. Current guidelines suggest that all patients with adult-onset epilepsy require imaging, ideally with MRI, unless an unequivocal diagnosis of idiopathic generalised epilepsy (which is not caused by a focal brain lesion) can be made.

An EEG can be extremely helpful if it is positive, although a normal interictal EEG certainly does not rule out the possibility of epilepsy. EEGs may be useful in determining seizure type (focal vs generalised) and risk of recurrence. The diagnostic yield of EEG abnormalities is greatest soon (<24 hours) after the event.

An ECG is cheap and easy and should be performed in all patients presenting with seizure, as cardiogenic syncope is a differential diagnosis.

What are the different types of seizures?

Seizures can be classified as:
- Partial (involving part of the brain)
- Generalised (involving the whole brain)

Partial seizures can be further classified as simple (with preservation of consciousness) or complex (with altered consciousness). Generalised seizures can be further clas-sified as idiopathic (with no underlying brain disease) and symptomatic (with associated brain disease or developmental delay). Table 7.2 gives examples of each type of seizure.

What issues does the treating doctor need to cover?

The diagnosis of a first seizure may be relatively straightforward, but the issues it raises can be extremely complicated. For this reason, it is ideal if patients can be referred to a first seizure clinic where all of these issues can be discussed.

Heather is referred to a first seizure clinic and has a list of questions for the doctor there.

'I've had one seizure. What are the chances I will have another one?'

The risk depends on whether the seizure was deemed to be provoked or not. A provoked seizure is one that is caused by an acute brain insult (e.g. hypoglycaemia, alcohol intoxication or withdrawal, subarachnoid haemorrhage, meningitis); if the provoking factor can be identified and withdrawn the risk of further events is low (around 3% for a reversible metabolic insult such as hypoglycaemia). It is higher (around 10%) if the provoking factor results in a structural brain lesion (e.g. ischaemic stroke).

Overall the risk of recurrence after an unprovoked first seizure is around 40%, although this varies enormously according to the type of seizure, based

Table 7.2 Classification of seizure types.

Partial		Generalised	
Simple – with retained consciousness	Complex – with clouding of consciousness	Idiopathic – no underlying neurological disorder	Symptomatic*– seizures occur secondary to underlying brain disorder
Unilateral limb jerking	Head-turning	Tonic-clonic seizures	
Unilateral sensory changes	Lip smacking	Classical absence	
	Automatisms (fidgeting, picking)	Myoclonic jerks	
	Preceding *déjà vu* or aura		

NB Partial seizures may progress to secondary generalisation. Secondary generalised seizures may be followed by focal neurological signs, e.g. Todd's paresis, a post-seizure unilateral limb weakness.

* Often associated with developmental delay.

on brain imaging and EEG results. The risk is greatest in the first 6 months; after 2 years the risk falls to <10%.

'Do I need to take medication?'

In general, patients with a first seizure are not started routinely on treatment unless they are judged to be at a particularly high risk of recurrence. The following factors increase the risk of recurrence and if they are present, treatment may be started after a single clinical episode:

• Previous history of other seizure types (e.g. myoclonic seizures, absences, partial seizures)
• Structural brain lesion
• Definite epileptic discharges on EEG
• If the patient or doctor considers the risk of a recurrent episode to be unacceptable

Because the treatment with antiepileptic drugs (AEDs) is long term and may be lifelong, and because each of

these drugs has potentially serious side effects, if there is any doubt about the diagnosis it is better to wait until there is certainty before committing the patient to a course of treatment that may be easy to start but less easy to withdraw from.

If a decision is made to use medication after the first seizure, or if the patient re-presents and a decision is made to start, the medication selected depends on the type of seizure and on its interactions with other drugs. In general:

• Generalised seizures are treated with sodium valproate, lamotrigine, levetiracetam or topiramate
• Partial (or partial-onset) seizures are treated with carbamazepine, topiramate or valproate
• Other agents used include gabapentin, clobazam and oxcarbazepine
• Different medications work for different patients
• Monotherapy is greatly preferable to combination therapy, which is indicated only in refractory seizures

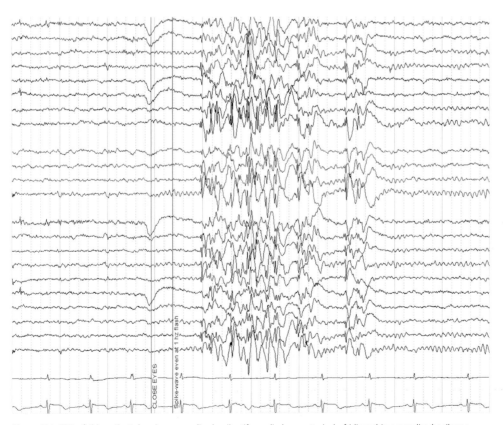

Figure 7.1 EEG of this patient showing generalised epileptiform discharges typical of idiopathic generalised epilepsy.

PART 2: CASES

'Can I drive? Can I work?'

The legal situation in the UK is that after an unprovoked seizure, drivers of cars or motorcycles should not drive for 6 months. It is the patient's duty to inform the relevant authorities and the treating doctor is not obliged to do so, although this is a possible course of action if the doctor believes that the patient is continuing to drive against medical advice. The restriction is longer (at least 10 years) for patients who are drivers of commercial vehicles.

Advice about work and hobbies depends on the patient's occupation; certain jobs would pose risks to the patient if they were to have a seizure whilst at work (e.g. scaffolder, heavy machinery operator). Negotiation should take place between doctor, patient and employer and if necessary the patient should be moved to alternative duties if this is possible.

'Will I pass it on to my children?'

The heritability of epilepsy depends very much on its underlying cause. Some forms are partly inherited (e.g. idiopathic generalised epilepsy), others occur as a consequence of some other condition (e.g. head injury, stroke) and are not strongly heritable.

There are specific implications of a diagnosis of epilepsy for women of childbearing age. Some anticonvulsant drugs (particularly sodium valproate) are associated with an increased risk of fetal malformations and should be avoided in women planning to become pregnant. Other anticonvulsants (e.g. carbamazepine) have enzyme-inducing effects and can therefore interact with the oral contraceptive pill, rendering it ineffective.

Heather has an EEG and attends the first seizure clinic. The EEG has shown generalised epileptiform discharges and the treating neurologist believes that she has idiopathic generalised epilepsy (Fig. 7.1). They discuss the pros and cons of starting treatment and she decides not to take medication at the present time. However, she re-presents with two further generalised seizures, and decides to start on medication with lamotrigine. She has no further seizures on medication and is able to return to driving after 2 years.

CASE REVIEW

This young woman presents with a witnessed loss of consciousness, and a diagnosis of first seizure is made. Many patients with a single seizure may never have a recurrent event, but in this case she went on to develop epilepsy. The type of seizure described and the EEG findings of generalised epileptiform discharges make it likely that she has idiopathic generalised epilepsy. The impact of this diagnosis on her lifestyle has to be considered, and specific issues apply to women of childbearing age in decisions about anticonvulsant treatment.

KEY POINTS

- A careful witness history is crucial in making a diagnosis of a seizure
- A single seizure is relatively common and most patients do not require treatment, unless they are judged to be at a high risk of recurrence
- Seizures can be classified as focal or generalised; focal seizures can be simple or complex and generalised epilepsies can be idiopathic or symptomatic
- In patients requiring medication, the choice of anticonvulsant depends upon the type of epilepsy (focal vs generalised), side effect profile, co-morbidities, and other medications being taken.

Further reading and references

Smith PE. Neurology in practice. The bare essentials: epilepsy. *Pract Neurol* 2008;**8**:195–202.

Case 8 A 30-year-old woman found fitting on the train

The ambulance paramedics rush into the emergency department with Jane Doe, an unidentified woman who looks to be around 30 years old, who was found convulsing on a railway train. She was alone in a carriage and has no identification on her person and no Medic-Alert bracelet. She was found lying on the floor shaking her arms and legs and making grunting noises by the guard. He knew what a seizure was because his daughter has epilepsy, and he phoned an ambulance immediately. However, they were a long way out of the station and it took 25 minutes for the train to return. She continued to convulse for the duration of the train journey and subsequent ambulance ride, despite the crew giving large doses of diazepam, and by the time she reached hospital had been fitting for over 40 minutes.

The emergency registrar attends to examine the patient, and finds a young woman, unresponsive, with eyes tightly closed and resisting eye opening. She was moving all four limbs in a bizarre and violent manner, rocking her body from side to side and flailing her limbs asynchronously. She did not respond to voice or to painful stimuli. Administration of intravenous diazepam reduced the movements slightly but she continued to shake. After several doses of diazepam, she began to snore and her oxygen saturations dropped and she had to be intubated and transferred to the intensive care unit.

What is the likely differential diagnosis?

The train guard and ambulance personnel have managed the patient as for status epilepticus (see Case 4). However, there are several features of the episode that are unusual for an epileptic seizure:

1 Long duration of attack: most seizures are short-lived and self-terminating within a few minutes. It is possible, however, for status epilepticus to be the first presentation

of epilepsy or other disorders of the nervous system such as meningitis or a structural lesion (see Cases 10 and 26).
2 Waxing and waning of movements: with the administration of diazepam, an epileptic seizure would often cease, or there might be no response at all; but in this patient's case it appeared to change in character.
3 Nature of movements: the limb movements do not sound typical of a generalised tonic-clonic seizure because the arms and legs are moving asynchronously and the body is rocking sideways. However, some types of frontal lobe seizure can produce bizarre, asynchronous movements of this sort.
4 Forced eye closure: this is unusual for an epileptic seizure. Typically the eyes would be open or the patient would not be able to resist the examiner's eye opening.

These features should alert the clinician to the possibility that this is not an epileptic seizure, and could be a pseudoseizure or non-epileptic attack (Table 8.1). In practice, differentiating a pseudoseizure from an epileptic seizure can be very difficult, even for experienced clinicians. Where there is doubt, it is safer to treat a patient for status epilepticus as this condition has a high mortality if untreated.

What are the key features of the history and examination?

The scenario of an unconscious patient who has no identifying documents is a challenging one in the emergency department. Ideally, we would like to know the following details urgently:

1 Is there a past medical history of epilepsy or other neurological problems?
2 Is the patient on any regular medications?
3 Is there a history of recent drug or alcohol ingestion?

In practice, it may not be possible to ascertain any of these facts, and management will have to be guided on the clinical examination.

Neurology: Clinical Cases Uncovered, 1st edition. © M. Macleod, M. Simpson and S. Pal. Published 2011 by Blackwell Publishing Ltd.

Table 8.1 Features of epileptic and non-epileptic seizures.

	Epilepsy	Non-epileptic attacks
Duration	Usually <2 minutes	Often prolonged
Motor features	Synchronised clonic movements	Asynchronous thrashing movements, may have side-to-side head or body movements, pelvic thrusting or rocking
Injury/tongue biting	Often	Sometimes
Recall afterwards	Almost never	Often preserved

The examination should concentrate on the following features:

1 Airway, breathing and circulation (as for any unwell patient).
2 Conscious level and Glasgow Coma Score.
3 Blood glucose level (in any patient with altered consciousness, this is essential).
4 Eye opening and pupillary responses.
5 Nature and distribution of the movements.
6 Reflexes and plantar responses.
7 Evidence of trauma sustained during the attack.

Jane Doe is taken to the intensive care unit with a ventilator to assist respiration. When the diazepam wears off, she begins to wake up, and the movements begin again. This time they last for only a few seconds at a time, stopping and starting. The ICU nurse notes that they get worse when she is attending to the patient, and seem to settle down after a while when Jane is left on her own. She calls the ICU doctor and asks whether they need to start a phenytoin infusion.

What is the appropriate treatment?

As outlined above, it is better to err on the side of treating a non-epileptic seizure as epilepsy, than vice versa. However, drugs such as phenytoin have undesirable side effects and administering them to patients who do not require them can be detrimental. If available, an urgent EEG could be performed during the event, and if it is normal while the patient is still having the attack it is reassuring to the clinician in the diagnosis of a non-epileptic seizure.

The ICU doctor is unable to get an urgent EEG as it is the middle of the night. He therefore decides to load the patient with phenytoin. This has no effect on her movements and she eventually has to be sedated with propofol. The neurology registrar attends to review the patient the following morning, and the sedation is removed. She continues to make abnormal movements. The neurology registrar feels that it is likely to be a pseudoseizure or non-epileptic attack, and the patient is subsequently extubated. The movements continue, but an EEG performed during the attack is entirely normal.

Later on that day, the patient's partner comes to hospital; he had had an argument with her the previous day and she had disappeared to the train station after that. He tells the treating doctors that she has been in three other hospitals in the city with the same problem over the previous year. She has also been unwell with abdominal pain, and is under investigation at a different hospital for asthma, but so far the tests have been all clear.

When he arrives, she wakes up and the movements stop. She discharges herself from hospital before any further interventions can be arranged, and does not attend for follow-up.

Non-epileptic attacks: what should we call them?

There are a multitude of different terms used for non-epileptic attacks, including:

• Pseudoseizures
• Hysterical attacks
• Dissociative attacks/seizures
• Non-epileptic attack disorder

Some of these are considered pejorative by some patients, as they may give the impression that the patients are deliberately 'faking it'. Terms which use the word 'seizure' may give a false impression that these events are epileptic, and should also be avoided. A neutral term, such as 'non-epileptic attack' or 'dissociative attack', is probably best for doctor and patient.

Who gets non-epileptic attacks?

Like other functional symptoms (see Case 12), non-epileptic attacks are thought to be an unconscious manifestation of psychological stress. Demographically, they are more common in women (75%), with onset usually in the late teens or twenties, and in 80% there is a history of other medically unexplained symptoms. Some research has shown that there are higher rates of previous abuse in patients with non-epileptic attacks and other functional disorders.

Sometimes patients with an EEG-confirmed definite diagnosis of epilepsy also have attacks which are non-epileptic. This is more common in patients with learning disability, and can pose a great challenge for diagnosis and treatment. However, it should be considered when attacks are completely resistant to drug treatment, and when withdrawal of medication leads to the re-emergence of another seizure type.

How do you diagnose non-epileptic attacks?

Diagnosis can be very difficult, and even experienced clinicians are sometimes mistaken. A study using videotapes of events that were shown to a specialist epileptologist compared to a gold standard of ictal video EEG (available in only a few centres), showed that the diagnosis was correct only 80% of the time. Diagnosing correctly is very important, however, as an incorrect label of epilepsy can result in lifelong treatment with anticonvulsant drugs, when in fact the therapy required is psychological.

How do you treat non-epileptic attacks?

As with other functional disorders, treatment begins with an explanation of the condition to the patient. It is important to emphasise to the patient that the doctor understands that the attacks are real, and that the patient is not 'making them up'. Regardless of their aetiology, frequent disturbances of consciousness are distressing to onlookers and disabling to the patient. It should be explained to the patient that the attacks are likely to be triggered by psychological stress, the cause of which may or may not be apparent to them, and that they are not 'crazy'. Non-epileptic attacks can be viewed as a maladaptive way of coping with psychological stressors; the patient 'switches off' from unpleasant thoughts or memories rather than having to confront these. Therefore identifying and addressing this underlying problem, usually in the form of counselling or psychotherapy, may be successful in treating the seizures. Once a definite diagnosis has been made, and if it is clear that the patient is having only non-epileptic events without coexisting seizures, any existing anticonvulsant medication can be withdrawn. However, this should be done slowly in case a withdrawal seizure is triggered.

CASE REVIEW

This patient presented as an emergency with a presumed diagnosis of status epilepticus. However, there were a number of features about the presentation that were atypical, and doctors were alerted to the possibility of a non-epileptic attack. These can be difficult to diagnose, and patients are often treated presumptively for epilepsy while investigations are being undertaken. The management of non-epileptic attacks is different from seizures, and involves psychological therapies and withdrawal of anticonvulsant medications; however, in some patients both types of attack may coexist.

KEY POINTS

- Distinguishing between epilepsy and non-epileptic attacks on clinical grounds can be difficult
- Where there is doubt, it is safer to treat for epilepsy rather than assume attacks are non-epileptic. In some patients, the two types of attack can coexist
- There are a number of clinical clues in the diagnosis of non-epileptic attacks
- Ictal video EEG is the gold standard for diagnosis but is not widely available
- Treatment consists of an adequate explanation to the patient, withdrawal of anticonvulsant medication, and psychological therapies

---

Further reading and references

Baker GA, Brooks JL, Goodfellow L, Bodde N, Aldenkamp A. Treatments for non-epileptic attack disorder. *Cochrane Database Syst Rev* 2007;Issue 1:CD006370.

Case 9 — A 66-year-old woman with confusion and weakness

Mrs Atkinson is a 66-year-old woman who presents to the emergency department at 10.10 am having been brought to hospital by ambulance. She seems to be having some difficulty in making herself understood, and is unable to give a clear account of what has happened. Unfortunately the ambulance crew have left the hospital on another call, and there is no information available on how she got to hospital.

What is the likely differential diagnosis?

This is very difficult in the absence of a history, and the differential diagnosis is wide. The priorities for medical care are to establish whether she is at any immediate risk (airway, breathing, circulation), to ensure she does not have a metabolic cause for her problems, to determine a clear history of what happened to her, and to determine the precise nature of her communication difficulties.

Possible causes might be categorised as due to: problems with the clarity of her thoughts (acute confusion, dementia, psychosis); aphasia (expressive or receptive aphasia due to involvement of cortical structures subserving language); problems with the muscular control of speech (dysarthria); problems with the generation of sound (aphonia); longstanding mutism; or elective (volitional) mutism.

She is breathing without difficulty or respiratory distress, has a pulse of 103 beats/min, which is irregularly irregular in time, force and volume, and has a blood pressure of 176/97 mmHg. She is apyrexial, with a capillary blood glucose of 6.4 mmol/L.

These findings suggest atrial fibrillation and hypertension. The atrial fibrillation might be a consequence of, for instance, a respiratory tract infection, which might in turn cause acute confusion through hypoxia or hyponatraemia. However, she is normothermic, which is somewhat against a systemic infection. Alternatively, the atrial fibrillation might instead be due to mitral valve disease, with confusion as a consequence of subacute bacterial endocarditis. Marantic (septic) embolism from an infected heart valve may have caused a cerebral abscess in the dominant hemisphere causing aphasia, or thrombus may have formed in the left atrial appendage as a result of relative blood stasis (due to the atrial fibrillation), with subsequent embolism to the dominant hemisphere and ischaemic stroke. Finally, she may have chronic atrial fibrillation and be on warfarin, and her communication difficulties, and indeed her hypertension, may be due to haemorrhage into her dominant left hemisphere.

Just then her daughter telephones the emergency department from another city some miles away, to enquire after her mother. You manage to speak to her on the phone, and she is clearly in some distress. She tells you her mother has previously enjoyed good health without hypertension or diabetes, and as far as she knows has never been on a tablet to thin her blood. Her mother worked as a shop assistant until her retirement 6 years ago, walks the dogs for half a mile each day and swims once a week. She last spoke to her mother 5 days ago, at which time she was well and had no complaints. She knows her mother is in hospital because a neighbour saw an ambulance outside the local newsagent and was shocked to discover who they had come for. Apparently her mother had come over 'all queer' while buying a pint of milk.

This information is very helpful, because for the first time we have some idea of what happened, and how quickly things developed. A week ago our patient was well, and as far as we can tell something quite dramatic happened quite quickly this morning. We can immediately exclude dementia and longstanding mutism. Acute confusion remains a possibility, and it is now something

Neurology: Clinical Cases Uncovered, 1st edition. © M. Macleod, M. Simpson and S. Pal. Published 2011 by Blackwell Publishing Ltd.

54

PART 2: CASES

of a priority to determine exactly what happened in the newsagent this morning.

> On telephoning the newsagent you learn that your patient was completely normal when she went in to the shop. Suddenly, at about 09.20 am, she appeared to be unsteady on her feet, she dropped her purse from her right hand, turned to speak to the shopkeeper but was able to say only 'dog … speak … help'. It is now 10.40 am.
>
> Initial neurological examination shows her to be alert but to have communication difficulties; she is able to obey one stage (stick out your tongue) but not three stage (point to the ceiling after pointing to the door) commands. The right side of her face is drooping, her right arm and leg lie flaccid at her side with no spontaneous movements, and she is able to move the left arm and leg briskly to command. She appears to have a right homonymous hemianopia.

The sudden onset now makes a stroke highly probable. Coma or headache do not appear to be salient parts of the history, and she is in atrial fibrillation of recent onset without anticoagulation. While an ischaemic stroke is a much more likely cause of her symptoms than a haemorrhagic stroke, this can only be confirmed by CT scanning. This distinction is crucial because if she has had an ischaemic stroke she is likely to benefit from thrombolysis with tissue plasminogen activator if treatment can be given within 4.5 hours of symptom onset.

Importantly, she has involvement of predominantly cortical functions (e.g. language) as well as motor function, and with the hemianopia this suggests a large volume of brain is involved. This is a total anterior circulation syndrome (TACS; Table 9.1), and without treatment her chances of disability-free survival are in the order of 5%. Clearly her condition now is substantially worse that at the onset, when only her language function appeared to have been involved. Fluctuation in the early stages of stroke is very common, improvement may not be sustained, and in her case it is likely that she has an occlusion of the left middle cerebral artery due to thromboembolism from a left atrial thrombus related to her atrial fibrillation.

> A CT brain scan has already been arranged and you arrange for a CT angiogram to be carried out at the same time and for both of these to be done immediately. The unenhanced CT shows no evidence of haemorrhage or of ischaemic change, but the CT angiogram shows occlusion of the left middle cerebral artery consistent with the presence of an occlusive thrombus (Fig. 9.1).

Table 9.1 OCSP (Oxfordshire Community Stroke Project) clinical classification of stroke.

Total anterior cerebral syndrome	Weakness and sensory loss of face arm and leg
	Homonymous hemianopia
	Expressive dysphasia (dominant hemisphere)
	Inattention (non-dominant hemisphere)
Partial anterior cerebral syndrome	Some but not all of above; must include at least one of homonymous hemianopia or relevant language or inattention deficit
Lacunar syndrome	Motor and/or sensory deficit without other features
Posterior circulation syndrome	Ataxia, nystagmus, nausea and vomiting
	Hemiparesis
	Cranial nerve signs
	May also include hemianopia and memory problems

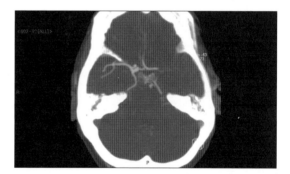

Figure 9.1 CT angiogram of the patient showing occlusion of the left middle cerebral artery.

The clinical salience of the pathophysiological processes that underlie stroke is that, in the early stages of stroke, neurological impairment (in this patient's case aphasia and right-sided hemiparesis) is due to neuronal dysfunction rather than irreversible death, but with the passage of time (usually a few hours) irreversible damage may occur. When blood flow returns within a short period, the neurological impairment usually resolves completely, and the episode is attributed to a transient ischaemic attack (TIA) (although these may be associated with

> ### Box 9.1 Pivotal systematic review
>
> Review: Thrombolysis for acute ischaemic stroke
> Comparison: 1 Any thrombolytic agent versus control
> Outcome: 17 Death or dependency by time to treatment up to 6 hours: rt-PA: all trials regardless of time window
>
> | Study or subgroup | Thrombolysis n/N | Control n/N | Peto Odds Ratio Peto,Fixed,95% CI | Weight | Peto Odds Ratio Peto,Fixed,95% CI |
> |---|---|---|---|---|---|
> | **1 Treatment within 3 hours** | | | | | |
> | NINDS 1995 | 155/312 | 192/312 | | 17.4% | 0.62 [0.45, 0.85] |
> | ECASS I 1995 | 28/49 | 25/38 | | 2.3% | 0.70 [0.29, 1.66] |
> | ECASS II 1998 | 39/81 | 44/77 | | 4.5% | 0.70 [0.37, 1.30] |
> | ATLANTIS B 1999 | 3/13 | 12/26 | | 1.0% | 0.39 [0.10, 1.49] |
> | ATLANTIS A 2000 | 7/10 | 7/12 | | 0.6% | 1.62 [0.29, 8.90] |
> | **Subtotal (95% CI)** | **465** | **465** | | **25.8%** | **0.64 [0.50, 0.83]** |
> | Total events: 232 (Thombolysis), 280 (Control) | | | | | |
> | Heterogeneity: Chi^2 = 1.83, df = 4 (P = 0.77); I^2 = 0.0% | | | | | |
> | Test for overall effect: Z = 3.34 (P = 0.00082) | | | | | |
> | **2 Treatment between 3-6 hours** | | | | | |
> | ECASS 1955 | 143/264 | 160/269 | | 14.8% | 0.81 [0.57, 1.13] |
> | ECASS II 1998 | 148/328 | 167/314 | | 18.1% | 0.72 [0.53, 0.99] |
> | ATLANTIS B 1999 | 133/284 | 128/286 | | 16.0% | 1.09 [0.78, 1.51] |
> | ATLANTIS A 2000 | 55/61 | 47/59 | | 1.7% | 2.26 [0.83, 6.14] |
> | EPITHET 2008 | 18/37 | 26/43 | | 2.3% | 0.62 [0.26, 1.50] |
> | ECASS 3 2008 | 140/418 | 155/403 | | 21.3% | 0.81 [0.61, 1.07] |
> | **Subtotal (95% CI)** | **1392** | **1374** | | **74.2%** | **0.85 [0.73, 0.99]** |
> | Total events: 637 (Thombolysis), 683 (Control) | | | | | |
> | Heterogeneity: Chi^2 = 7.57, df = 5 (P = 0.18); I^2 = 3.4% | | | | | |
> | Test for overall effect: Z = 2.06 (P = 0.039) | | | | | |
> | **Total (95% CI)** | **1857** | **1839** | | **100.0%** | **0.79 [0.69, 0.90]** |
> | Total events: 869 (Thombolysis), 963 (Control) | | | | | |
> | Heterogeneity: Chi^2 = 12.77, df = 10 (P = 0.24); I^2 = 22% | | | | | |
> | Test for overall effect: Z = 3.47 (P = 0.00051) | | | | | |
> | Test for subgroup differences: Chi^2 = 3.37, df = 1 (P = 0.07), I^2 = 70% | | | | | |
>
> 0.1 0.2 0.5 1 2 5 10
> Favours thombolysis — Favours control
>
> This Forrest plot shows the results from seven randomised controlled trials in acute stroke involving 3696 patients. The squares represent the best estimate of effect of tissue plasminogen activator (tPA) on death and dependency in the individual studies, and the horizontal bars the 95% confidence limits in each study; the black diamonds show the overall effect for: (1) treatment within 3 hours, (2) treatment started between 3 and 6 hours after stroke onset, and (3) for the overall dataset. A poor outcome was seen in 232/465 (50%) of patients treated with tPA within 3 hours compared with 280/465 (60%) in the control group, and overall in 869/1857 (47%) of tPA-treated patients and 963/1839 (52%) of controls. (From Wardlaw *et al.* 2009.)

MRI evidence of permanent structural brain damage). Early reinstatement of blood flow is an important therapeutic approach in stroke, and intravenous treatment with the clot-busting drug tissue plasminogen activator (tPA) is effective if given within the first 4.5 hours. Efficacy at later time points, and with intra-arterial approaches to reperfusion, is the subject of ongoing clinical trials. The clinical definition of TIA is that symptoms and signs should resolve completely within 24 hours, and this has dictated that some patients will be treated with tPA whose symptoms may have been due to a TIA and would have resolved spontaneously. However, these patients were included in clinical trials of tPA, and so efficacy in patients with continuing neurological impairment at the time of treatment is well established (Box 9.1).

Other evidence-based treatments for acute ischaemic stroke include management in an acute stroke unit, immediate initiation of antiplatelet therapy with aspirin, and, for selected patients with hemispheric stroke and reduced consciousness, decompressive hemicraniectomy (Table 9.2).

Table 9.2 Evidence-based treatments for acute ischaemic stroke.

Intervention	Proportion of patients likely to be eligible	Number needed to treat to prevent one death/disability	Net benefit per 1000 stroke patients
Stroke unit care	80%	26	31
Acute aspirin	50%	83	6
Intravenous thrombolysis	15%	18	8
Decompressive hemicraniectomy	1%	4	4

Mrs Atkinson receives intravenous thrombolysis with tPA beginning at 11.20 am. By 13.00 there has been some improvement in her right-sided weakness, and by that evening her speech has also improved.

What next?

Mrs Atkinson was transferred to a stroke unit as soon as the tPA infusion was complete, and she should continue to be managed, and receive rehabilitation, in that environment. Her known atrial fibrillation might be the cause of her stroke, but it is important to exclude significant narrowing in the left internal carotid artery (she might benefit from end arterectomy) or valvular heart disease. Her atrial fibrillation puts her at substantial increased risk of recurrent stroke, and this risk can be substantially reduced by anticoagulation, for instance with warfarin. However, the optimum timing for the introduction of warfarin is not clear; for a patient like Mrs Atkinson – with what has been a substantial volume of brain injured – it is usual to have the patient on aspirin, starting 48 hours after the tPA, and to introduce warfarin 2–3 weeks later. There is no well evidenced role for heparin in this setting.

Further reading and references

Donnan GA, Fisher M, Macleod M, Davis SM. Stroke. *Lancet* 2008;**371**:1612–23.

van der Worp HB, van Gijn J. Clinical practice. Acute ischemic stroke. *N Engl J Med* 2007;**357**(6):572–9.

Wardlaw JM, Murray V, Berge E, del Zoppo GJ. Thrombolysis for acute ischaemic stroke. *Cochrane Database Syst Rev* 2009; Issue 4:CD000213. DOI: 10.1002/14651858.CD000213.pub2.

CASE REVIEW

This patient with atrial fibrillation and hypertension presented with confusion and the sudden onset of speech problems and a right-sided weakness. Her confusion was due to aphasia, and she was unable to give an account of herself. Using corroborative sources of history (the daughter, her friend and the newsagent) it was possible to make a secure diagnosis, to allow the institution of appropriate treatments.

KEY POINTS

- Patients with dysphasia may at first assessment appear to be confused
- In those with communication difficulties (e.g. aphasia) or who were unconscious at the time of the attack (e.g. epilepsy), a corroborative source of history, even by telephone, can be invaluable
- Because thrombolysis is such an effective treatment, knowing with precision the time of onset can be crucial in being able to deliver such treatments
- Stroke severity can be assessed using simple clinical scales, and these can provide important guides to prognosis

PART 2: CASES

Case 10 An 18-year-old girl with headache, fever and confusion

Amanda Wright, an 18-year-old A-level student has been brought into her local accident and emergency department one lunchtime by her parents who have become extremely concerned about her. As you take a history from Amanda, it becomes apparent she has difficulty paying attention to what is going on around her; she is clearly in some discomfort and keeps trying to roll away under the covers. Her parents report that Amanda has been complaining of feeling 'feverish' and 'headachy' since getting up that morning. She has been sick three times. Her symptoms were initially attributed to a migraine but she has become increasingly drowsy and irritable as the day has progressed with symptoms of word finding difficulties and apparent confusion with disorientation.

Routine observations include a temperature of 38.9°C, blood pressure of 90/60 mmHg, a pulse of 100 beats/min and oxygen saturations of 98% on room air.

What is the likely differential diagnosis?

The presentation of headache and vomiting in a young woman is most commonly due to migraine, but in this case the drowsiness and pyrexia mean that other causes must be sought and if possible ruled out. In a young person with a short history of headache, meningism, confusion and speech difficulties, metabolic, toxic and infective aetiologies need to be considered. This includes bacterial, viral and atypical infections of the central nervous system, acute renal or hepatic failure, and potential toxic effects of prescribed or recreational drugs. More rarely, an inflammatory or neoplastic cause may be responsible such as a cerebral vasculitis, systemic lupus erythematosus or leukaemia. Her rapid deterioration over the past 12 hours is a sinister sign and investigations and further management need to be conducted swiftly.

Neurology: Clinical Cases Uncovered, 1st edition. © M. Macleod, M. Simpson and S. Pal. Published 2011 by Blackwell Publishing Ltd.

Further history reveals that Amanda has been previously fit and well and takes no regular medications. She has been performing well in her recent coursework and has been offered a place at university to study physiotherapy. Amanda lives with her parents and younger sister Sheila, and no one else in the family has been unwell. She does not smoke, drinks approximately 6 glasses of wine a week, and there is no history of recreational drug use. There is no history of recent foreign travel.

On examination, her Glasgow Coma Scale score is 13/15 (eyes open to speech (3), confused speech (4), obeys motor commands (6)). Her Mini-Mental State Examination score is 21/30 with deficits in orientation, attention and calculation, memory and naming. Some more detailed testing reveals difficulties with spontaneous speech, comprehension, reading and writing. There is no evidence of a skin rash. She has neck stiffness on passive neck flexion. Her pupils are equal and reactive to light and the fundi appear normal. There is a full range of extraocular movements. The remainder of the cranial nerve examination is unremarkable. Tone is normal in the limbs and power full in all muscle groups. Reflexes are present and symmetrical with bilateral downgoing plantars. There are no cerebellar signs.

What would you do next?

Amanda's clinical state is clearly deteriorating rapidly. The first step is to ensure her airway, breathing and circulation are adequately maintained and supplemental oxygen and intravenous fluids are given as required.

What tests would you consider performing?

Investigations must rapidly exclude an infective meningitis (inflammation of the meninges) or encephalitis (inflammation of the brain parenchyma), as well as potential metabolic and toxic causes of her symptoms. Blood samples should be taken for full blood count, urea and electrolytes, liver function tests, glucose, blood cultures, erythrocyte sedimentation rate and C-reactive protein. A chest X-ray will exclude an associated chest infection. A CT or MRI scan of the head should be performed to rule out cerebral oedema with raised intracranial pressure or a mass lesion. In encephalitis there may be changes consistent with oedema around the temporal lobe or orbitofrontal gyri. A lumbar puncture should be performed to investigate for changes in the cerebrospinal fluid consistent with bacterial or viral infection.

Which organisms are commonly responsible for bacterial meningitis in adults and how would you treat Amanda to cover for bacterial infections?

The common bacteria causing infection in adults are *Streptococcus pneumoniae*, *Neisseria meningitidis* and *Haemophilus influenzae*. Bacterial meningitis is a medical emergency. Delay in treatment increases mortality and morbidity and if the diagnosis is suspected intravenous treatment with broad-spectrum antibiotics such as ceftriaxone should be started immediately, without delay for tests such as scans or lumbar puncture. *Listeria monocytogenes* infection may arise in immunocompromised individuals and the elderly and may be treated by ampicillin and gentamicin; it has limited sensitivity to ceftriaxone. Meningococcal meningitis can evolve rapidly with fulminant septicaemia, meningitis, fever, hypotension, development of a petechial or purpuric rash, rapid deterioration in conscious level and neck stiffness. Amanda is pyrexial, confused, drowsy and hypotensive with neck stiffness. Her symptoms have progressed rapidly and antibiotic treatment should be started immediately and continued until an alternative diagnosis has been confirmed or the treatment is complete.

> Amanda's investigations include normal urea and electrolytes, liver function tests, glucose, erythrocyte sedimentation rate and C-reactive protein. Her full blood count showed an elevated white cell count (18 × 10^9/L) with predominant neutrophilia.
>
> A lumbar puncture demonstrated an opening pressure of 32 cmCSF (<20 cmCSF) which was turbid. She had 3200 white cells/mm^3 (85% neutrophils), 200 red cells/mm^3, a protein of 2.3 g/L (<0.45 g/L) and a CSF glucose of 1.2 mmol/L (serum glucose 6.0 mmol/L). Microscopy demonstrated Gram-positive cocci. A sample was sent for polymerase chain reaction studies including for herpes simplex 1 and 2, Ebstein–Barr virus, varicella zoster virus, cytomegalovirus, pneumococcus and meningococcus as well as tuberculosis.

How do you interpret these CSF findings?

The CSF is turbid with a high opening pressure, elevated protein, reduced glucose and a markedly elevated white cell count with neutrophilia. These results in conjunction with the clinical history support a diagnosis of bacterial meningitis such as caused by meningococcus or *Strep. pneumoniae* (Table 10.1).

How would you treat Amanda?

She has already been started on ceftriaxone, and this should be continued while awaiting formal bacteriological identification and drug sensitivities. Intravenous treatment should continue for at least 7 days. If aciclovir has previously been started this can now be stopped. Systematic review and meta-analysis suggests that corticosteroids improve outcome and reduce the risk of neurological sequelae in both children and adults, so unless there is a contraindication they should be used.

Which other infections need to be considered if Amanda had been travelling abroad recently?

Herpes encephalitis can cause a very similar clinical presentation, but these CSF findings are very much in favour of a bacterial meningitis. The same holds for Japanese B encephalitis, spread by the *Culcine* mosquito endemic in India and Asia. This virus affects the basal ganglia and thalamus causing tremor and Parkinsonian features. There is no specific treatment but the virus may be prevented by vaccination. A related virus causes western Nile virus in North America. Cerebral malaria should always be considered in returning foreign travellers. This can be diagnosed by thick and thin blood films.

> That evening the bacteriology lab telephoned to report that the CSF ELISA (enzyme-linked immunosorbent assay) was positive for Strep. pnemoniae, and the following day they rang again to say that culture was also positive, with full sensitivity to ceftriaxone.

What is Amanda's prognosis?

The prognosis in bacterial meningitis depends crucially on the delay to initiation of treatment. In this case, where presentation has been rapid with immediate initiation of antibiotic therapy, mortality is low and the vast majority of patients make a full recovery.

PART 2: CASES

Table 10.1 Typical CSF findings in bacterial and viral meningitis.

	Opening pressure	Appearance	Protein (g/L)	Glucose (mmol/L)	White cell count (10^9/L)	Red cell count (10^9/L)
Migraine	<25 cmCSF	Clear	May be modest elevation	Normal	<10	<10
Venous sinus thrombosis	Elevated	Clear	Elevated	Normal	<10	<10
Bacterial meningitis	Elevated	Turbid	Elevated	Reduced	>1000	<100
Bacterial meningitis (treated)	May be elevated	May be turbid	May be elevated	Reduced	>50	<100
Viral meningitis	May be elevated	Clear	May be elevated	Reduced	May be elevated	<100, unless haemorrhagic
Subarachnoid haemorrhage	May be elevated	Bloodstained	Elevated	Reduced	1/1000 of red cell count	>500
Idiopathic intracranial hypertension	Elevated	Clear	Normal	Normal	<2	<10
Tuberculous meningitis	Elevated	May be turbid	Elevated	Reduced	10–200	<10
Normal	<20 cmCSF	Gin clear	<0.44	4–10 mM	<2	<10

Amanda was discharged home after receiving 2 weeks of intravenous antibiotics and making a good symptomatic recovery. By 4 weeks she had no residual neurological symptoms or signs but was troubled by overwhelming fatigue on minimal exertion; by 6 months this too had resolved.

CASE REVIEW

This female presented with a short history of headache, meningism, drowsiness and disorientation. Both her level of consciousness and her cognitive function were impaired, and prior to treatment she was deteriorating rapidly. The initial CSF findings are highly suggestive of bacterial meningitis, and the diagnosis was later confirmed by ELISA and CSF culture. With appropriate treatment rapidly instituted she went on to make a good recovery.

Further reading and references

van de Beek D, de Gans J, Spanjaard L, Weisfelt M, Reitsma JB, Vermeulen M. Clinical features and prognostic factors in adults with bacterial meningitis. *N Engl J Med* 2004;**351**(18): 1849–59.

KEY POINTS

- Rapidly progressing symptoms of confusion, fever and speech disturbance in a young patient may be due to infective, toxic, metabolic or vascular causes and need to be investigated urgently
- If a bacterial or viral infection of the central nervous system is suspected clinically, appropriate treatment should be administered rapidly, and should not be delayed whilst investigations – such as CT or lumbar puncture – are awaited
- Routine blood tests, blood cultures and lumbar puncture may all provide useful diagnostic information in viral encephalitis
- Intravenous antibiotics are extremely effective in treating bacterial meningitis if treatment is initiated early
- As with many acute disturbances of cerebral function, while there may be a rapid recovery and resolution of symptoms and signs, the patients may be left with non-specific problems such as fatigue, and these may persist for some months

A 30-year-old woman with double vision and fatigue

Arlene is a 30-year-old teacher who makes an appointment to see her GP because of double vision. She has noticed this intermittently for the past month or so, particularly when she is watching television after a hard day at work. She has been feeling generally tired, and has had to stop her evening netball sessions because she has been too tired. Things are now so bad that she has difficulty climbing the three flights of stairs to her flat. She is feeling short of breath on minimal exertion. At work, she is having difficulty because her voice is becoming hoarse towards the end of lessons. She went on the internet and wonders if her thyroid needs to be checked.

What is the likely differential diagnosis?

Arlene describes a number of symptoms that are non-specific (fatigue and lethargy) but also symptoms that raise the suspicion of a neurological disease (diplopia and hoarse voice). The decrease in exercise tolerance may simply represent fatigue, but may signify neurological muscle weakness affecting either the limbs or the respiratory muscles.

The generalised nature of the symptoms (which involve the eyes, voice, limb muscles and possibly respiratory muscles) would suggest a diffuse process. This is far more likely to be a lower motor neuron lesion, affecting peripheral nerves, muscles or the neuromuscular junction. However, a multifocal process affecting the central nervous system is also a possibility. Further history and examination are required to differentiate these possibilities.

What are the key features of the history and examination?

The neurologist should clarify the symptoms further by asking the following:

Neurology: Clinical Cases Uncovered, 1st edition. © M. Macleod, M. Simpson and S. Pal. Published 2011 by Blackwell Publishing Ltd.

1 Are there any sensory symptoms and what is their distribution? Disturbances of sensation would suggest a problem in the peripheral nerves, brain or spinal cord and would argue against a disease of the muscle or neuromuscular junction. However, muscle pain may be a feature of the inflammatory myopathies.

2 What is the pattern of weakness throughout the day and how is it affected by exercise? Lesions of the neuromuscular junction, and specifically myasthenia gravis, are associated with fatigability – weakness which typically worsens throughout the day and is exacerbated by exercise. For example, patients may complain of hoarseness that worsens towards the end of a telephone conversation, or difficulty chewing towards the end of a meal. Primary muscle diseases may be associated with worsening weakness on exercise, and with muscle pain associated with activity.

3 Is there weakness of the bulbar or respiratory muscles? It is important to ask about dysphagia (difficulty swallowing), choking (and whether on liquids or solids), dysphonia and dysarthria. These are symptoms of a bulbar palsy, and can indicate that patients are at risk of aspiration secondary to ineffective swallowing mechanisms. Involvement of the muscles of speech and swallowing can also indicate potential involvement of the respiratory muscles; therefore it is important to assess respiratory function during the clinical assessment.

4 What is the nature of the visual disturbance? Double vision can also result from lesions in various sites of the nervous system. It is important to try and ascertain whether the double vision is fixed or variable, and whether it occurs only in some positions of gaze (which may suggest an individual cranial nerve palsy) or whether it is more generalised. It is also important to ask about eye pain, loss of acuity or loss of colour vision, which are all symptoms of optic neuropathy and may be confused with 'double vision'.

The clinical examination should assess the following:

1 Eye movements: are the eye movements abnormal, and if so do they fall into the distribution of one or more cranial nerves? If not, this may be a complex ophthalmoplegia, which can occur with diseases of the neuromuscular junction as well as with thyroid ophthalmopathy and metabolic disturbance such as Wernicke's encephalopathy.

2 Pupils: pupillary reactions should be normal in disease of the neuromuscular junction.

3 Eyelids: ptosis may be subtle and is often associated with the ophthalmopathy of myasthenia.

4 Is there dysarthria or dysphonia, or palatal weakness? As mentioned above, these are signs of a bulbar palsy. It is also important to look for associated weakness of neck flexion, which can be a predictor of respiratory muscle involvement.

5 Are there sensory changes? The presence of sensory abnormalities argues against myopathy or neuromuscular junction disease and suggests a peripheral neuropathy or central nervous system pathology.

6 Are the reflexes normal? Again, reflexes should be normal in myopathy (unless there is extensive muscle wasting) or neuromuscular junction disease.

7 Is there clinical evidence of thyrotoxicosis or hypothyroidism? These are both differential diagnoses in the history above.

8 Is there evidence of other autoimmune disease (e.g. vitiligo, Addison's disease, rheumatoid arthritis, lupus)? These have an association with myasthenia gravis.

9 Is there fatigability? This can be assessed in various ways depending on the muscle involved:
  • Ptosis: fatigability can be demonstrated by asking the patient to look up for a sustained period, after which the ptosis may be more pronounced
  • Dysphonia/dysarthria: ask the patient to speak for a prolonged period, e.g. 'count to a hundred' and assess whether the dysphonia is worse afterwards
  • Limb weakness: test muscle strength before and after exercise (e.g. climbing stairs, or making 'chicken wing' movements with the arms); a decrease in strength is highly suggestive of myasthenia

10 Is there respiratory muscle involvement? This is crucially important and requires a vital capacity meter (not a peak flow meter). Patients with neuromuscular respiratory weakness may be at risk of requiring ventilatory support.

Arlene has a number of abnormal findings on examination. She has bilateral ptosis, which is fatigable, and double vision in all planes of gaze with difficulty looking laterally in both directions and impaired vertical gaze. Her pupils and visual fields are normal. Her speech initially appears normal, but towards the end of the consultation she is slurring some words and her voice appears softer. She has normal limb strength on pre-exercise testing but bilateral weakness of shoulder abduction to 4/5 after exercise. Sensory examination and reflexes are normal. Her vital capacity is within normal limits.

The examination findings suggest a complex ophthalmoplegia, with diplopia and abnormalities of eye movement, which do not fall into the distribution of any individual cranial nerve. This is associated with fatigability affecting the speech and the limb power. This combination of findings is highly suggestive of a disorder of the neuromuscular junction.

What investigations are required?

On the basis of the history and examination, the most likely diagnosis is myasthenia gravis. This is an autoimmune disease where antibodies are formed against the acetylcholine receptor at the neuromuscular junction, which impedes transmission across the synapse (Fig. 11.1b). Table 11.1 summarises the other varieties of neuromuscular junction disease. Different patterns of weakness are produced; some patients have generalised myasthenia, others have symptoms confined to the eyes or to speech and swallowing (oculobulbar myasthenia). Subsequent investigations are aimed at confirming the diagnosis and ruling out the differentials. The patient requires the following:

1 Blood test for acetylcholine receptor antibodies (positive in 85% of patients with generalised myasthenia and 50% of patients with isolated ocular myasthenia) or anti-muscle specific kinase (MUSK) antibodies (present in 40–50% of patients with negative acetylcholine receptor antibodies).

2 Blood tests should also be performed for thyroid function (which can cause lethargy and diplopia), full blood count and routine biochemistry (anaemia or metabolic disturbance can cause lethargy and shortness of breath).

3 Spirometry for vital capacity to assess respiratory muscle function (see Case 3 on Guillain–Barré syndrome).

4 Where acetylcholine receptor antibodies are not present, electrophysiological testing including repetitive stimulation and single fibre electromyography (EMG)

study can be helpful (the latter is positive in 90% of patients with myasthenia).

5 Where acetylcholine receptor antibodies are not present and electrophysiological testing is equivocal, a tensilon test (administration of a short-acting cholinesterase inhibitor, which increases the amount of acetylcholine at the neuromuscular junction and should improve transmission) may be indicated. Where positive, it is very helpful, but it may be equivocal and requires a definite endpoint (e.g. ptosis, weakness) that can be measured before and after administration of the drug. Bradycardia can be a side effect of tensilon and therefore the drug should be given where appropriate resuscitation facilities are available.

6 CT scan of thorax: 75% of patients have an abnormality of the thymus gland, which may be either hyperplasia or a malignant thymoma, in which case surgical removal is required.

What is the treatment?

Once the diagnosis is made, myasthenia is treated using a combination of symptomatic and disease-modifying therapy summarised in Table 11.2. Most patients require a combination of treatments (Fig. 11.1c,d). In some

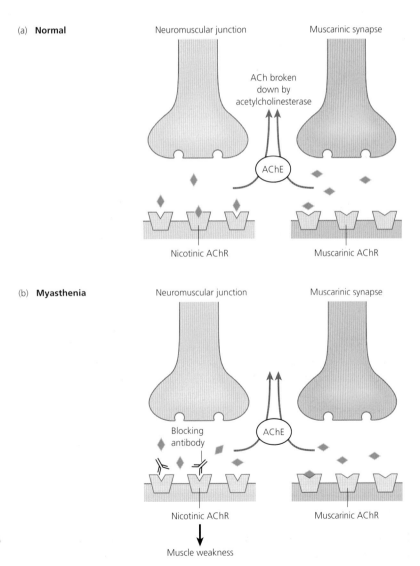

(a) **Normal**

Neuromuscular junction   Muscarinic synapse

ACh broken down by acetylcholinesterase

AChE

Nicotinic AChR   Muscarinic AChR

(b) **Myasthenia**

Neuromuscular junction   Muscarinic synapse

Blocking antibody

AChE

Nicotinic AChR   Muscarinic AChR

Muscle weakness

Figure 11.1 Normal transmission across the neuromuscular junction (a) and in myasthenia gravis (b).

PART 2: CASES

(c) **Following treatment with cholinesterase inhibitor (pyridostigmine)**

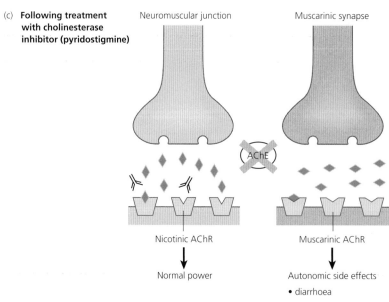

(d) **Following treatment with cholinesterase inhibitor and muscarinic antagonist (propantheline)**

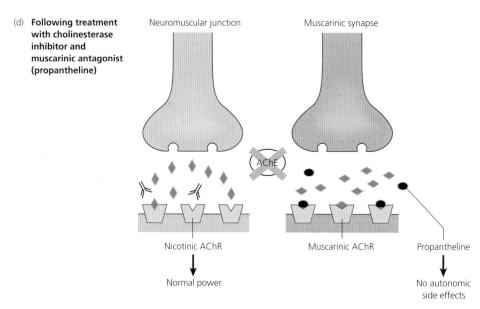

Figure 11.1 (*Continued*) (c, d) The effect of different drug treatments in myasthenia. AChE, acetylcholinesterase; AChR, acetylcholine receptor.

Table 11.1 Diseases of the neuromuscular junction.

Disease	Characteristics	Antibody	Per cent positive
Myasthenia gravis (generalised)	Diplopia, ptosis, dysarthria, fatigable limb weakness +/– respiratory muscle weakness	Acetylcholine receptor (AChR) or anti-MUSK	90% 50% if AChR –ve
Myasthenia gravis (ocular/bulbar form)	Any age, female predominance Diplopia, ptosis, dysarthria	Acetylcholine receptor	50%
Lambert–Eaton myasthenic syndrome	Proximal leg weakness, later arm weakness, ptosis. Seldom bulbar involvement or diplopia 50% have cancer (small cell lung cancer)	Voltage gated calcium channel	95%
Botulism	Rapid progression, bulbar and eye muscles	None	–
Congenital myasthenic syndromes	Family history, no response to myasthenia drugs, antibody negative, childhood onset	None	–
Drug-induced myasthenia	History of treatment with penicillamine or (rarely) statins	None	–

Table 11.2 Drug treatment of myasthenia gravis.

Drug class	Example	Mechanism
Cholinesterase inhibitor	Pyridostigmine	Replacement of acetylcholine at the neuromuscular junction: symptomatic therapy
Immunosuppressants	Prednisolone Azathioprine (steroid-sparing) Mycophenylate mofetil	Decrease production of antibodies: disease-modifying therapy

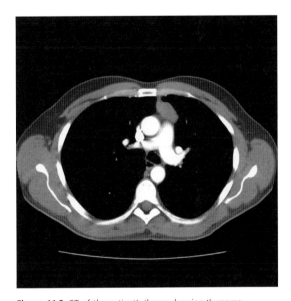

Figure 11.2 CT of the patient's thorax showing thymoma.

patients who are refractory to these immunosuppressants, additional possibilities include cyclosporine or methotrexate. In patients who are rapidly worsening (so-called myasthenic crisis) or refractory to the above therapies, intravenous immunoglobulin or plasma exchange may be required, and sometimes ICU care is necessary for respiratory support.

Patients with a thymoma may require thymectomy to prevent local spread, sometimes with adjuvant radiotherapy. Some patients with myasthenia without a thymoma may also benefit from thymectomy in terms of improved disease control.

Arlene underwent several investigations including a tensilon test (which was positive) and antibody testing, which confirmed the diagnosis of myasthenia gravis. She was commenced on treatment with pyridostigmine and her symptoms improved markedly. A CT scan of the thorax (Fig. 11.2) showed a thymoma and she underwent surgery. Her myasthenia subsequently remitted and she was able to stop therapy after 2 years.

PART 2: CASES

CASE REVIEW

This patient presents with a history of fatigable weakness affecting the limbs and oculobulbar muscles. This combination of symptoms is highly suggestive of a disease of the neuromuscular junction, the most common of which is myasthenia gravis. She was diagnosed by tensilon test and electrophysiology, and commenced on treatment which included acetylcholinesterase inhibitors, immunosuppression and thymectomy, and had a good outcome. Myasthenia may recur in later life, or may develop *de novo* in older people and should not be forgotten about in the elderly.

KEY POINTS

- Myasthenia gravis is an important cause of generalised weakness, ophthalmoplegia and a bulbar palsy, which can occur in all age groups
- The symptoms can be non-specific and it may be mistaken for a functional disorder
- Respiratory muscle involvement can be severe and require ventilatory support; vital capacity should be monitored
- Diagnosis is made clinically with supportive evidence from EMG, antibody assay and the tensilon test

Further reading and references

Hilton-Jones D. How to do it: diagnose myasthenia gravis. *Pract Neurol* 2002;**2**:173–7.

Thanvi B, Lo T. Update on myasthenia gravis. *Postgrad Med J* 2004;**80**(950):690–700.

Case 12 A 29-year-old woman with tingling weakness of the left arm and leg

Case 12   A 29-year-old woman with tingling weakness of the left arm and leg

Mary Carrone, a 29-year-old right-handed policewoman, presented to the accident and emergency department with left-sided weakness and tingling. She is worried she is having a stroke.

What are the key features of the history?

When did her symptoms start, how have they evolved, are they constant or intermittent, and if intermittent, how long do they last?

She was first troubled with her symptoms about 4 weeks ago, when she noticed a left-sided tingling numbness while lying in bed one night. She describes her left arm feeling as if she's been lying on it and it had 'gone to sleep'. She didn't think very much of it and it only lasted a few minutes. Over the following weeks the tingling numbness returned, intermittently, with each episode seeming to last longer than the last, until 2 weeks previously when she reports that the numbness became constant, at least to some extent all of the time. Her symptoms began to become intrusive, in that whereas previously she would just continue about her business, she now found that she was distracted from what she was trying to do and becoming worried as to the cause of these symptoms.

Since then she has also noticed that the left hand appears to have become weaker; she has difficulty holding a kettle or a heavy pan, and has difficulty transferring her young son from his pram to his car seat. Because of her symptoms she has been moved to office-based work, and she has found that she is much slower on the keyboard than usual. Over the last few days her symptoms have been getting worse to the extent that she attended A&E because she thought she was having a stroke.

Neurology: Clinical Cases Uncovered, 1st edition. © M. Macleod, M. Simpson and S. Pal. Published 2011 by Blackwell Publishing Ltd.

What other features of the history are important?

1 What are the associated symptoms?
   • Palpitations, chest tightness, choking sensation, difficulty getting breath or angor animi (extreme distress with a fear of impending doom)
   • Tingling around the mouth and tongue
   • Sense of derealisation or depersonalisation
   • Headache; visual or speech disturbance; nausea, vomiting, photophobia or phonophobia
2 What are the possible triggers of this episode?
   • What was she doing when the symptoms came on
   • Have there been recent stressors or life events
   • Have there been remote stressors or life events
3 Does she have any relevant past medical history?
   • Have there been previous episodes of neurological dysfunction
   • Is there a past history of depression, anxiety or panic attacks
   • Is there a history of migraine, irritable bowel syndrome, hysterectomy, endometriosis, non-ulcer dyspepsia, fibromyalgia or chronic fatigue syndrome

She says that at the beginning there were no associated symptoms, and all she had was the tingling numbness. However, as time has gone on she finds increasingly that her symptoms have periods when they are much worse, and that at these times she feels unwell in herself, with shortness of breath, a feeling that she is chocking for air, and tingling all over including her lips and tongue. Sometimes she feels separated from reality, as if observing herself from outside. For the last 2 weeks she has had a constant headache, and she finds that even ordinary daylight hurts her eyes.

She lives with her partner and three children aged 5, 3 and 13 months. They have no financial worries, but her mother recently died after a long battle with breast cancer complicated in the later stages by cerebral metastases;

during the last months of her life she was able to stay at home, and Mary was her main carer.

There is no personal or family history of migraine. Mary has had no previous episodes of neurological dysfunction or of panic attacks, but she did have a short episode of postnatal depression after the birth of her second child. There is no history of irritable bowel syndrome, hysterectomy, endometriosis, non-ulcer dyspepsia, fibromyalgia or chronic fatigue syndrome. However, as a child she experienced recurrent episodes of abdominal pain and ear infections which resulted in substantial hospital contacts.

What is the likely differential diagnosis?

This is a complicated history, and requires careful analysis; her symptoms cannot be attributed to a lesion at a single anatomical site. The left-sided symptoms might be due to right hemisphere dysfunction (e.g. migraine, demyelination, low-grade glioma, venous infarction, ischaemic stroke), to a cervical radiculopathy or to carpal tunnel syndrome. The speed of onset and the duration is not typical of ischaemic stroke and the duration is not typical of migraine. None of these diagnoses account for the breathing difficulties, the circumoral paraesthesia or the derealisation, which are more typical of panic or anxiety attacks.

There are therefore three possible explanations for her symptoms: they might all be explained by organic disease, or not at all explained by organic disease, or they might be due to a combination of an initial organic disease exacerbated by an emotional or psychological response to the fear that this has engendered.

Rarely, a low-grade glioma in the temporal lobe can give rise to seizures with contralateral sensory disturbance and associated symptoms of anxiety. However, one would expect these symptoms to be intermittent rather than continuous, to have developed over a longer period, and perhaps to have been associated with more obvious manifestations of a seizure disorder.

Sensory symptoms as described here, with a rapid escalation over a short period of time and with associated symptoms of panic are most likely be a manifestation of a functional or non-organic neurological problem. Supporting evidence includes the recent loss of her mother, the history of postnatal depression and her unexplained abdominal pain as a child. Frequently, such problems arise in the context of a relatively trivial problem such as an attack of migraine. Importantly, symptoms not explained by organic disease are no more

under the control of the sufferer and no less disabling than symptoms caused by organic disease.

What are the key features of the examination?

The primary purpose of the examination is to seek objective evidence of impairment of neurological function, such as might be caused by a right hemisphere or peripheral nerve lesion as described above. The characteristic features of a pyramidal weakness with brisk left-sided reflexes and an upgoing left plantar response are of more diagnostic value than objective reports of altered sensory perception in response to light touch or pin prick sensation. Similarly, globally brisk reflexes, particularly in the absence of upgoing plantars, are seldom of significance. Patients may manifest a 'give way' weakness, where they are able to generate full power for brief periods and then the power 'collapses'.

In addition, it is sometimes the case that a patient is unable to generate full power when asked directly, but is able to do so when their focus is elsewhere; for example, a patient who is able to walk must have power of at least 4/5 in the legs in spite of what might appear to be the case on the couch. Hoover's sign is present when there is weakness of hip extension – in this case on the left – on direct testing, but normal power of left hip extension when testing flexion of the right hip, and is highly suggestive of a functional, rather than a structural, neurological problem.

Examination showed an inconsistent, variable weakness of the left arm. Reflexes were very brisk in that arm, but were also brisk in the right arm and in the legs. Plantars were symmetrically downgoing. She reported that both cottonwool and pin prick stimulation felt 'different' in the left face, arm and leg, but acknowledged that she could feel that she was being touched. Hoover's sign was negative.

How should patients with functional neurological problems be managed?
Investigation

The decision as to whether, and how much, to investigate such patients will depend to a very large extent on the patient's own fears and wishes. When the clinical scenario is typical (as here), investigation is not required. While many patients will be very happy to accept the explanation offered and will be relieved that they do not have an irreversible neurological problem, others may still harbour doubt, and may question whether a doctor can tell such things just by examining them.

In such cases, or where there is a degree of diagnostic uncertainty (such as where there have been previous episodes of disturbed neurological function suggestive of multiple sclerosis), it is reasonable to request brain imaging, most helpfully an MRI scan. However, the patient should understand that this is being done explicitly to rule out diagnoses such as low-grade glioma, and that there is a possibility that it may demonstrate incidental variations from normal (e.g. chiari malformation, unruptured aneurysms) that might have implications for their health but for which the prognosis, and optimal management, are not clearly known.

Treatment

1 *Psychological support and therapy.* Sometimes patients develop functional neurological problems in the context of obvious stressors, perhaps with associated symptoms of depression. They should be offered help and support from, for instance, a liaison psychiatrist or a psychologist to allow them to explore the issues surrounding their presentation, and to receive drug treatment for depression if this is indicated. Where patients present with functional neurological problems without obvious recent stressful events, it may be either that their symptoms will remain medically and psychologically unexplained, or that they have their genesis in deeper more longstanding stressors. These might include domestic violence or sexual abuse and – particularly where the patient or others might still be at risk – it is important to give the patient the opportunity to disclose this in a caring, confidential and supportive environment.

2 *Physical therapy.* Just because the neurological impairment does not have an identifiable cause does not mean that it is not troublesome for the patient, and equally does not mean that physical therapies directed at maximising function and minimising impairment (predominantly physiotherapy and occupational therapy) do not have an important role in promoting recovery, and these should be offered.

3 *Organisation of treatment.* Ideally, both psychological and physical therapies should be delivered by members of the same multidisciplinary team. This will allow consistency of approach and explanation, and the development of a comprehensive programme of cognitive behavioural therapy and a programme for the gradual and paced return to normal activities.

CASE REVIEW

This woman presented with a subacute onset of predominantly sensory, initially intermittent, symptoms affecting the left side of the body. As time progressed these became associated with symptoms of panic disorder. While she felt her sensation was clearly affected, the remainder of the examination was essentially normal. The likelihood is that these symptoms are functional, and while a confident clinical diagnosis can be made in cases such as these, in practice patients usually have an MRI arranged before they see a neurologist.

KEY POINTS

- Remember that every speciality has its share of medically unexplained diseases, and neurology is no exception
- Not every patient with a functional weakness has a history of irritable bowel syndrome, myalgic encephalomyelitis, fibromyalgia, non-ulcer dyspepsia and depression
- While some patients are able to identify a recent source of stress or worry which has provoked the onset of their weakness, this is not usually the case
- Rather than 'putting patients' minds at rest', continuing investigation and involvement with health services often leads to increased health-related anxiety

Further reading and references

Stone J. The bare essentials: functional symptoms in neurology. *Pract Neurol* 2009;**9**:179–89.

Case 13 A 45-year-old woman with pain in the leg

Jeannie, a 45-year-old secretary, has made an appointment with her GP to get a sick note for work; she normally keeps well, but the past month has been troubled by terrible pains down her right leg. She has real trouble sitting at a desk all day, and using the foot pedals for the audio typing machine is causing her great discomfort.

What are the key features of the history?

1 What is the site of the pain and does it radiate anywhere?
  • Is there back pain
  • What is the distribution of pain in the leg
  • Does it radiate down into the feet or up into the buttocks
2 What is the character of the pain?
  • Shooting and shock-like
  • Dull, aching and pressure-like
3 What is the duration of symptoms and how does the pain alter over the course of the day?
4 Are there any 'red flag' symptoms of bowel or bladder disturbance?
  • Urinary retention, frequency, urgency, incontinence
  • Constipation, faecal incontinence, loss of sensation
5 Is there any sensory loss in the legs, or any motor weakness?
6 Is there any history of trauma or surgery to the back or hips?
7 How severe is the pain and what functional limitations does it cause?

Jeannie first noticed the pain about 6 weeks ago, but it has been constant for more or less a month. She is aware of a dull ache in her back but the thing that really troubles her is

the pain shooting down her right leg, which feels like an electric shock. It goes all the way down the front of her leg to the top of the foot, and she is sometimes aware of pain in the buttocks, particularly on the right. It comes and goes during the day, and is worst at night in bed, or when she is driving, or at her desk with the foot pedals. It is really getting her down, and she is tearful as she talks about it. She has been constipated, but thinks that is because of the painkillers she has been taking (which have not really helped so far), but denies any bladder symptoms. She has difficulty walking because of the pain. There is no history of surgery or trauma, and she has never had similar symptoms in the past. She lives alone with her dog Rudolf, is a non-smoker and never drinks alcohol.

Where is the lesion and what are the key features of the examination?

Jeannie's symptoms affect only her right leg and are associated with back pain. In theory, this could be caused by a lesion in any of the following sites:
• Cerebral cortex (left hemisphere)
• Brainstem
• Spinal cord
• Nerve root
• Lumbar plexus
• Peripheral nerve

The nature of the symptoms (i.e. shooting pains, without motor weakness) would be most consistent with a lesion in the nerve root or plexus. However, partial spinal cord pathology would also be a possibility. Lesions in the cortex or brainstem would be more likely to affect the right arm in addition to the leg, and are therefore less likely. The absence of bowel and bladder symptoms would also argue against a spinal cord lesion.

The clinical examination should confirm that only the right leg is involved and that neither the right arm nor the left leg are involved (either of these features would dramatically alter the site of the lesion). It should also

Neurology: Clinical Cases Uncovered, 1st edition. © M. Macleod, M. Simpson and S. Pal. Published 2011 by Blackwell Publishing Ltd.

Table 13.1 Signs of lower and upper motor neuron lesions.

Lower motor neuron signs	Upper motor neuron signs
Decreased/normal tone	Increased tone
Muscle wasting	Pyramidal pattern of weakness
Fasciculations	Brisk reflexes
Loss of reflexes	Altered sensation in central distribution
Altered sensation in distribution of peripheral nerve or root	

> **Box 13.1 Causes of lumbar radicular pain/sciatica**
>
> - Lumbar disc herniation (commonest cause in young patients)
> - Spinal canal stenosis (commoner cause in the elderly)
> - Tumour infiltration
> - Infection (bacterial, viral)
> - Vascular malformations

> **!RED FLAG**
>
> - Motor weakness
> - Bowel or bladder involvement
> - Bilateral symptoms
> - History of malignancy
> - Acute onset of symptoms, particularly if associated with trauma or vascular disease

differentiate an upper motor neuron lesion (affecting cortex, brainstem or spinal cord) from a lower motor neuron lesion (root, plexus or peripheral nerve) (Table 13.1).

> On examination, she is overweight (110 kg) and looks depressed, but general medical examination is otherwise unremarkable. She has an antalgic gait with obvious discomfort on walking and on bending down. Examination of the cranial nerves and upper limbs is completely normal. In the lower limbs, tone, power and coordination are normal. She describes shooting pains down her right leg but there is no objective sensory loss to light touch, pin prick, temperature, vibration or proprioception. Straight leg raising is normal on the left but on the right is markedly reduced to 30° and reproduces the pain exactly. The reflexes are all present with reinforcement and the plantars are bilaterally downgoing.

What is the likely diagnosis?

Jeannie's symptoms are suggestive of a lower motor neuron lesion that affects the whole of the right leg. There is pain and altered sensation without motor weakness, and the reflexes are not brisk. Straight leg raising reproduces the symptoms. Therefore, the lesion is likely to be in the sensory root or dorsal root ganglion in the lumbar region. This is suggestive of the syndrome of lumbar radicular pain, commonly known as sciatica, which can have a variety of underlying causes (Box 13.1). There are no 'hard' neurological signs and no motor weakness or other 'red flag' symptoms to raise the strong possibility of any other condition.

What investigations are required?

Sciatica has a favourable natural history; with simple analgesics, most patients can expect a rapid and dramatic reduction in symptoms. For this reason, early imaging (to exclude other causes) is generally not indicated unless any of the following apply:
- 'Red flag' symptoms suggestive of other pathology
- Recurrent sciatica
- No resolution of symptoms after 4–6 weeks
- History of malignancy
- If surgery is being considered

In patients who do require imaging, MRI is the most appropriate test as it has the best resolution in the region of interest. Nerve conduction studies are generally not indicated.

What is the treatment?

Patients who do not respond to conservative treatment after several months and who are severely disabled by neurological symptoms should be considered for surgery. It is important to realise that the surgery will not improve back pain *per se*, but only the associated leg pains that go along with it.

An alternative to surgery is epidural steroid injection, although no clinical trials have convincingly demonstrated its efficacy, and the benefits may be only temporary.

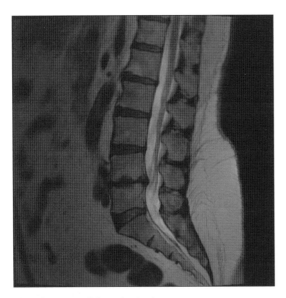

Figure 13.1 MRI of the patient's spine.

Jeannie's symptoms continued for more than 2 months, and began to get worse and to stop her sleeping at night. Her doctor requested an MRI of the spine (Fig. 13.1) which showed a small bulging disc. Given her obesity, the risks of surgery were felt to be high, and she was managed conservatively with analgesics and physiotherapy. She soon realised that she loved the treadmill in the gym, and began attending every day before work. She began to lose weight (a total of 35 kg), and as she did so her symptoms continued to improve. She began to walk her dog Rudolf every evening before dinner, and eventually struck up a firm friendship with Alfred, a 50-year-old man who had lost his wife a few years ago and was out walking his Alsatian. She quit her job and started her own business manufacturing handmade greetings cards. She remains pain-free 10 years later.

CASE REVIEW

This patient presents with back pain and shooting pains radiating down the leg without any signs or symptoms suggestive of other pathology. The diagnosis of sciatica is confirmed and other pathologies are ruled out by the clinical history and subsequent MRI findings. The patient improves with conservative management.

KEY POINTS

- Sciatica or lumbar radicular pain is a common condition and causes significant morbidity, but in the majority of cases is not associated with serious pathology
- Most cases resolve with conservative management
- Spinal imaging is indicated in patients who have 'red flag' symptoms suggestive of other pathology
- Surgery is reserved for patients who are not improving after conservative management and appropriate spinal imaging; it may improve symptoms in the legs but back pain alone is not a sufficient indication, even if severe

Further reading and references

Koes BW, van Tulder MW, Peul WC. Diagnosis and treatment of sciatica. *BMJ* 2007;**334**(7607):1313–17.

Case 14 A 29-year-old woman thrown from her horse

Sarah Tremlett is a 29-year-old solicitor who is brought into the accident and emergency department by ambulance after being thrown off her horse whilst riding. Sarah fell sideways and fell head first onto the ground; she was wearing a helmet at the time. Immediately after falling, she was able to speak to onlookers and although she was dazed, her eyes were open, she knew where she was and she complained of pain over the back of her head. Paramedics report that her conscious level dipped on the way into hospital. On assessment at the time of arrival in A&E by nursing staff, Sarah is unable to follow commands, her eyes are closed and only open when painful stimuli are administered above her eyes or over her sternum and she is making mumbling noises which make no sense. Her arms and legs withdraw away from painful stimuli. You are paged to come and assess her.

What should you do in the immediate assessment?

Immediate assessment of a trauma patient with a head injury often seems frantic, with rapid resuscitation, history-taking and examination all occurring simultaneously. This means an organised approach is essential to ensure that the assessment of the severity of head injury can be complete. Initial assessment begins with evaluation of airway, breathing and circulation.

Airway and breathing

Sarah's respiratory rate is 18 breaths/min. Her oxygen saturations are 99% on 4L of oxygen.

Paramedics should already have immobilised Sarah's spine and her neck should not be manipulated until a cervical fracture has been excluded. Indications for endotracheal intubation include depressed level of con-

Neurology: Clinical Cases Uncovered, 1st edition. © M. Macleod, M. Simpson and S. Pal. Published 2011 by Blackwell Publishing Ltd.

sciousness, respiratory distress (high respiratory rate and shallow breathing) or respiratory depression.

Circulation

Sarah's heart rate is 62 beats/min and blood pressure is 148/90 mmHg.

Tachycardia and hypotension may arise from shock as a consequence of bleeding into the thorax, abdomen and retroperitoneum, or tissues surrounding a long bone fracture. Sarah should, therefore, be examined for external signs of trauma to the neck, chest, abdomen and limbs.

Spinal shock can arise as a result of cord injury and results from acute loss of sympathetic outflow. Hypertension associated with a wide pulse pressure and bradycardia is termed Cushing's reflex and may be a sign of raised intracranial pressure.

A witness account of events is crucial. Concussion is common following a head injury with temporary loss of consciousness occurring at the time of impact. It is usually associated with a short period of amnesia.

On examination, there are no palpable fractures over Sarah's skull although there is a large haematoma above her right ear.

What was Sarah's conscious level immediately after falling and what is her conscious level now?

Almost all patients with life-threatening head injuries will have a depressed level of consciousness. Conscious level should be assessed using the Glasgow Coma Scale (GCS) (Box 14.1). This clinical rating scale quantifies eye opening (E) and verbal (V) and motor (M) responses to verbal and noxious stimuli in a reproducible manner and also allows changes in a patient's conscious level to be charted over time.

The lowest GCS score possible is 3/15 and the highest is 15/15. Coma is defined by the absence of verbal or

Box 14.1 The Glasgow Coma Scale.

	Patient response	Score
Eye opening	Spontaneous	4
	To speech	3
	To pain	2
	None	1
Best verbal response	Orientated	5
	Confused	4
	Inappropriate words	3
	Incomprehensible sounds	2
	None	1
Best motor response	Obeys commands	6
	Localises to pain	5
	Normal flexion	4
	Abnormal flexion	3
	Extends to pain	2
	None	1

complex motor responses to any stimulus and a GCS score of 8 or lower is frequently used to define coma.

Immediately after falling, Sarah's GCS score was 15/15 score (E3, V4, M5) and her GCS score is currently 8/15 (E2, V2, M4) indicating coma.

If a patient's conscious level allows it, further tests of mental status should be performed including tests of attention and concentration (subtracting serial 7s), orientation (to time, place and situation) and memory. Retrograde amnesia can be tested for by asking the last thing remembered prior to the injury and anterograde amnesia by asking about the first thing remembered after the injury.

Sarah's pupils are equal and reactive to light. Both sides of her face grimace when pressure is placed in the supraorbital regions on the left and right. Although she is unable to respond to commands, all four limbs flex in response to painful stimuli. Her tone appears normal although reflexes are brisker on the right and her right plantar is upgoing.

What is the severity of Sarah's head injury?
Head injury can be classified as minimal, moderate or severe, with risks of a poor outcome, and optimal management differs depending on the severity.

1 *High risk group:*
- GCS 3–8
- Major focal deficit
- Progressive decline in conscious level
- Depressed or penetrating skull fracture
2 *Moderate risk group:*
- GCS 9–14
- Minor focal deficit
- Vomiting
- Seizures
- Amnesia
- Major external trauma
3 *Minimal risk group:*
- GCS 15
- No focal neurological deficits
- No concussion

Sarah's conscious level and focal right-sided neurological signs place her in the high risk group.

What investigations are required?
All patients with traumatic injury above the level of the clavicles should have cervical spine films to rule out a fracture. Before a cervical collar can be removed, the cervical spine must be completely cleared from C1 to C7.

Routine blood tests include full blood count, urea and electrolytes, clotting profile and group and save.

Sarah's conscious level appears to have deteriorated since the time of impact. What diagnoses would you be concerned about in particular?
Her rapidly deteriorating conscious level and localising signs suggest an expanding subdural or extradural haematoma.

How would you investigate further for this?
A CT of the head should be performed looking for extradural and subdural blood. In addition a CT will identify:
- Subarachnoid and intraventricular blood
- Parenchymal contusions and haemorrhages
- Cerebral oedema
- Effacement of the perimesencephalic cisterns
- Midline shift
- Skull fractures and air–fluid levels

Due to her deteriorating conscious level, Sarah was intubated and ventilated prior to transfer to the CT scanner. Figure 14.1 shows one of the images that were obtained.

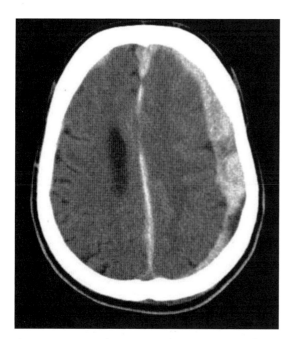

Figure 14.1 CT scan of the patient, demonstrating subdural haematoma and contusions.

associated with a short period of amnesia. The majority of patients with concussion have normal neuroimaging.

2 *Extradural haematoma:* extradural bleeding usually results from a tear in the middle meningeal artery. Approximately 75% of such cases are associated with a skull fracture. The typical clinical course proceeds from immediate loss of consciousness to a lucid interval, which is followed by a secondary depression in conscious level as the extradural blood expands. Progression to herniation and death can occur rapidly because the haematoma arises from an arterial bleed.

3 *Skull fractures:* these are important markers of potentially serious intracranial injury but they rarely cause symptoms themselves. If the scalp is lacerated over the fracture, it is considered an open, or compound, fracture. Linear fractures account for the majority of skull fractures and can usually be managed conservatively. Basilar skull fractures occur with more serious trauma and are frequently missed on routine skull films. These fractures may be associated with cranial nerve injury or CSF leakage from the nose or ear. Comminuted and depressed fractures are often associated with contusions of the underlying brain and require surgical debridement.

What is Sarah's diagnosis?

The CT images demonstrate the presence of a subdural haematoma and parenchymal contusions.

Subdural bleeding usually arises from a venous source with blood filling the space between the dural and arachnoid membranes. CT scanning usually reveals a crescentic collection of blood across the entire hemispheric convexity. Elderly and alcoholic patients are particularly prone to subarachnoid bleeding. In these groups of patients, large haematomas can result from trivial impacts or from acceleration/deceleration injuries such as whiplash injuries. Cerebral contusions are similar to 'bruising' of the brain as it moves across the inner surface of the skull. The inferior frontal and temporal lobes are the common sites of traumatic contusion. With lateral forces, contusions can occur just deep to the site of impact, or at the opposite pole as the brain impacts on the inner table of the skull. Contusions frequently evolve into larger lesions over 12–24 hours.

What are the other important potential consequences of traumatic head injury?

1 *Concussion:* this refers to a temporary loss of consciousness that occurs at the time of impact. It is usually

What action should you take next in Sarah's management?

The clinical assessment and CT scan suggest a severe head injury. An immediate referral should be made to neurosurgery at this point. If the decision is made to operate, surgery should proceed immediately because delays increase the likelihood of further brain damage during the waiting period.

What other criteria are considered when deciding whether or not to admit patients to hospital after a head injury?

All patients with symptoms of significant confusion, agitation or depressed consciousness should be admitted to a high-dependency ward for investigation and observation as should patients with new focal neurological signs or intracranial blood or fracture identified on a CT head scan.

Sarah was assessed by neurosurgeons and taken to theatre where her subdural haematoma was successfully evacuated. She was transferred postoperatively to the ICU department.

PART 2: CASES

What steps can be taken in Sarah's medical management at this point?

In general, patients like Sarah who have depressed conscious level should be intubated for airway protection. Placement of an arterial line allows accurate haemodynamic monitoring of blood pressure. Intracranial pressure (ICP) may be monitored by placement of an ICP monitor. The following measures should also be considered:

- Careful fluid management
- Nutritional support
- Temperature management
- Deep vein thrombosis (DVT) prophylaxis: at least in the first instance this should involve graduated compression stockings rather than anticoagulation
- Prophylaxis against gastric ulcers
- Treatment of post-truamatic seizures with anticonvulsants
- Further brain imaging (CT) if there is a significant deterioration in her clinical condition (usually by 2 or more GCS points sustained for 30 minutes, or a precipitous rise in ICP if this is being measured)

What is Sarah's prognosis?

The outcome after head injury is often a matter of great concern for patients with serious injuries. The admission GCS score has significant prognostic value. Patients scoring 3 or 4 have an 85% chance of dying or remaining in a vegetative state, whereas these outcomes occur in only 5–10% of patients with a score of 12 or higher. Postconcussion syndrome is common and results in a chronic profile of headache, fatigue, dizziness, difficulties concentrating, irritability and personality changes.

> *Sarah made an excellent postoperative recovery. Following a period of inpatient rehabilitation she was discharged and eventually returned to work and also to riding.*

CASE REVIEW

This woman fell from a horse, landed on her head, and initially seemed to be alright. However, soon afterwards she began to lose consciousness and by the time of hospital admission she had a GCS score of 8 and was at high risk of death or disability. The right upgoing plantar suggests a left hemisphere injury, and a CT scan of the brain confirmed a left subdural haematoma with underlying contusions to the brain. With appropriate neurosurgical intervention and rehabilitation she went on to make an excellent recovery.

KEY POINTS

- The GCS is an essential tool in the management of patients with head injury
- Detecting a falling GCS following head injury is crucial in identifying those patients who may benefit from prompt neurosurgical intervention
- Remember that low or high speed trauma may be associated with damage elsewhere (e.g. fractured spine, ruptured spleen) and vice versa; the patient with two fractured femurs following a road traffic accident may also develop an extradural haematoma while in hospital
- Good outcome following head injury depends on prompt assessment, early discussion with and transfer to neurosurgery, and the availability of a brain injury rehabilitation service

Further reading and references

Maas AI, Stocchetti N, Bullock R. Moderate and severe traumatic brain injury in adults. *Lancet Neurol* 2008;7(8): 728–41.

A 67-year-old man who is unsteady on his feet

Peter Davidson is a 67-year-old butcher who presented to his general practitioner because he had noticed that he was becoming increasingly unsteady on his feet and had fallen on two occasions in the last 6 months, most recently giving himself a black eye in the process. His GP refers him to the local neurology clinic for assessment of his unsteady gait.

What are the key features of the history?

1 How long has he been unsteady, and is the problem of sudden onset or gradually progressive?

2 Is his unsteadiness accompanied by feelings of giddiness or dizziness?

3 Why does he think he falls? Does he lose balance, lose muscle power, lose consciousness, stumble?

4 Does he go down in a heap or like a tree trunk?

5 What are the associated symptoms?
- Problems with articulation – dysarthria
- Problems with coordination in the hands (limb ataxia)
- Double vision or jumping vision
- Light-headedness, giddiness, presyncope
- Slowness and stiffness of movement
- Tremor
- Autonomic disturbance

6 Is there anything in the background history that might be important?
- Alcohol intake
- Drugs with cerebellar side effects – anticonvulsants
- Drugs with cardiovascular side effects – antihypertensives, drugs slowing the heart
- Drugs with extrapyramidal side effects – neuroleptics
- Smoking history
- Weight loss

Neurology: Clinical Cases Uncovered, 1st edition. © M. Macleod, M. Simpson and S. Pal. Published 2011 by Blackwell Publishing Ltd.

His symptoms have been apparent for the last 2 years, but in retrospect his wife says he was 'slowing up' for a few years before that. His two falls have occurred in daylight. The first happened when he was out getting the newspapers, when he seemed to trip over a ridge in a pavement and fell his length. The second occurred in the house, when he appeared to trip over the loose edge of a carpet in the hall, and struck his head on a telephone table as he fell. There was no loss of consciousness with his falls, and the power in his legs doesn't seem to fail him; rather, it is as if he stumbles and is unable to react quickly enough to stop himself, going down like a tree rather than crumpling in a heap. There are no symptoms of unsteadiness, giddiness or light-headedness. He reports no dysarthria, although his wife says the power of his voice is less than it was. There in no double vision or jumping vision (oscillopsia). He does find it increasingly difficult to use his hands, but this is more due to them being stiff, weak and tremulous rather than to clumsiness or incoordination. There is no bladder or bowel disturbance or disturbance of erectile function but he does report symptoms of light-headedness coming on within 15 seconds of rising from a seated position and persisting for perhaps 15 seconds thereafter. He has not experienced these symptoms at the time of his falls. He neither smokes nor consumes significant amounts of alcohol, and is not on any regular medications. There is no history of weight loss.

What is the likely differential diagnosis?

The differential diagnosis is that of impaired walking and falls in the elderly. In essence this can be categorised as problems with: (1) loss of consciousness; (2) awareness of and accounting for the environment (such as with poor vision, poor lighting, confusion); (3) the power required to remain upright (such as with proximal myopathy or stroke); or (4) the coordination of movement (such as with cerebellar or extrapyramidal problems).

In his case, it is clear from his and his wife's account that there is no loss of consciousness and no confusion, and his vision is reported to be normal. Specifically, there is nothing in the history to suggest the prodromal symptoms associated with reduced cerebral perfusion (giddiness, dizziness, light-headedness, sounds fading into the distance, sweating, nausea, vomiting, pallor reported by witnesses, palpitations) such as might be experienced with postural hypotension or a cardiac arrhythmia. In fact, he is clear that he does experience symptoms of postural hypotension at other times, but not at the time of his falls.

Weakness is not a predominant feature in the history and there is no weight loss, so predominantly motor causes such as stroke, myopathy or motor neuron disease are unlikely. So we are left with either a cerebellar disturbance or an extrapyramidal disorder.

Against a cerebellar disorder is the lack of associated symptoms such as clumsiness in the arms, double vision or jumping vision, or dysarthria. He does not drink and is not on any medications, so a toxic cerebellar disorder is unlikely; he does not smoke so a paraneoplastic cerebellar degeneration is unlikely. In contrast, there are features of an extrapyramidal disorder including progressive slowing of gait, loss of righting reflexes, bradykinesia, loss of manual dexterity and tremor.

What are the examination findings for extrapyramidal disorders?

The most telling part of the examination is the gait: patients are slow to rise from a chair and slow to move. Sometimes they find it very difficult to initiate walking movements (problems with gait ignition). Their stride length is shortened, they seem to shuffle forward with their weight in front of them (festination), they often have reduced arm swing, usually worse on one side than the other, and when they turn round they again take a number of small steps as if counting off the hours. When they stand still they have truncal rigidity and instability, in that if they are tugged backwards they may take a series of very small steps attempting to right themselves.

In the arms there is often (but not always) a fine resting tremor as if rolling a pill between the thumb and forefinger (a 'pill-rolling' tremor), sometimes also involving pronation and supination at the wrist. Typically this tremor is improved by action. The consequences of this tremulousness in the context of increased tone is a so-called 'cogwheel' rigidity, best elicited at the wrist or elbow and often made more apparent by asking the patient to move the contralateral limb (synkinesis). In the face there is often reduced facial expression, and increased sweating and salivation.

Box 15.1 Characteristic features of extrapyramidal disorders

Parkinson's disease	Asymmetrical onset, bradykinesia, tremor, postural instability, therapeutic response to L-DOPA
Multiple system atrophy	Associated autonomic symptoms, cerebellar signs, pyramidal signs
Progressive supranuclear palsy	Early falls (especially backwards), supranuclear gaze palsy, rigidity, dysarthria, dysphagia
Drug-induced Parkinson's disease	History of dopamine antagonist use (central: neuroleptic; peripheral: antiemetic), symmetrical symptoms and signs
Vascular Parkinson's disease	Gait affected much more than arms, tremor may be completely absent

---

Our patient walked up the corridor to the consulting with a stooped gait, reduced arm swing in the right arm, taking small steps, and appearing to freeze as he came into the examination room. He had axial rigidity, retropulsion and poverty of facial expression. He had a fine pill-rolling tremor of the right hand with increased tone in the right arm and to a lesser extent in the left arm, with associated cogwheel rigidity.

It seems highly likely that Peter has an extrapyramidal disorder, and the clinical features are typical of Parkinson's disease (PD). Characteristic features of other extrapyramidal disorders are given in Box 15.1.

What are the causes of extrapyramidal disorders?

The extrapyramidal system comprises overlapping circuits of information processing and involves the cortex, striatum, globus pallidus, thalamic and subthalamic nuclei and the substantia nigra. Important components are the dopaminergic neurons whose cell bodies lie in the substantia nigra and whose axons project to the striatum. Extrapyramidal disorders are usually due to: (1) deficiencies in dopamine signalling due to neurodegenerative disease affecting the dopaminergic cells of the substantia nigra (not enough dopamine released); (2) antagonism of the action of dopamine at its receptor by dopamine antagonists such as chlorpromazine; or (3) loss of postsynaptic dopamine target cells due to their degeneration (such as in multiple system atrophy or progressive supranuclear palsy). Other causes of Parkinsonism include small vessel cerebrovascular disease ('vascular Parkinsonism'). In a small proportion of cases, PD is inherited, with defects in over 16 genes described.

How should patients with Parkinson's disease be managed?
Drug treatment
There are no treatments that alter the underlying neurodegenerative process that causes PD. Treatment strategies are therefore based almost entirely on manipulating neurotransmitter, particularly dopaminergic, signalling (Fig. 15.1). Broadly, this might be achieved through using direct dopamine agonists (such as ropinirole or pramipexol); by increasing the availability of the dopamine precursor L-dihydroxy-phenylalanine (L-DOPA; as co-careldopa or co-beneldopa); or by preventing the breakdown of dopamine (by inhibiting monoamine oxidase (MAO) or catechol-O-methyl transferase (COMT)). This is relatively complicated, because dopamine has peripheral effects including nausea and vomiting, abdominal pain and diarrhoea, vasoconstriction and hypertension. Treatments must therefore increases central dopaminergic signalling without substantially increasing peripheral signalling. This may be achieved either by co-treatment with a dopamine antagonist that is unable to penetrate the blood–brain barrier or, in the case of L-DOPA therapy, by inhibiting, in the periphery only, the enzyme that converts L-DOPA to dopamine, again using a drug that does not cross the blood–brain barrier.

A further complication is that treatment effectiveness declines over time, and it seems that at least some of this change is not due to progression of the underlying disease. Normally, synaptic dopamine levels are high following depolarisation of the presynaptic membrane but then fall rapidly under the influence of MAO and COMT. In PD, treatments can lead to a constantly high synaptic concentration of dopamine, and it appears that over the years this in itself can modulate the extrapyramidal system with the emergence of unpredictable side effects as circulating dopamine levels rise following dosing, reach their peak, and then fall.

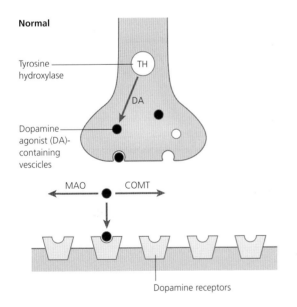
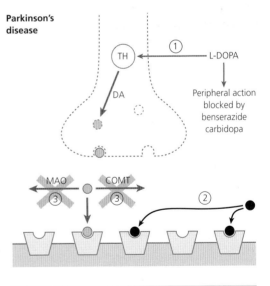

① L-DOPA increases endogenous dopamine production in surviving neuron

② Direct dopamine agonists (e.g. ropinirole) increase transmission

③ Inhibitors at COMT (entacapone) or MAO (selegiline) increase the availability of dopamine in the synaptic cleft

Figure 15.1 Basis of drug treatment in Parkinson's disease.

Most troublesome of these effects are the L-DOPA-induced dyskinesias, which often emerge after 5–10 years on L-DOPA therapy and which can prove very difficult to manage. This is one rationale for the practice of initiating treatment with dopamine agonists in younger patients in order to delay the onset of L DOPA-induced dyskinesia. However, it is not clear that, for a given intensity of dopaminergic therapy, they are any less likely to induce dyskinesias than are L-DOPA-containing preparations.

One important side effect of dopamine agonism, of which patients should be warned, is impulsivity with poor impulse control, which can lead to uncharacteristic and inappropriate behaviours including altered sexual behaviours and financial recklessness.

Non motor complications of Parkinson's disease can be more difficult to treat and include cognitive and behavioural problems, sleep disturbances, pain and autonomic dysfunction leading to symptomatic postural hypotension.

Surgery

For patients with refractory disease or with very troublesome dyskinesias, it has been suggested that deep brain stimulation directed at the subthalamic nuclei or transplantation of fetal dopaminergic cells may convey some benefit. However, while deep brain stimulation is offered in some centres, the proportion of patients who have access to and might benefit from these interventions is small; and there is as yet insufficient evidence of efficacy for stem cell therapies to be recommended outside clinical trials.

Organisation of care

As with other chronic and progressive neurological conditions, much of the challenge lies not in the treating of the underlying illness but rather in: (1) the provision of support to maintain functional independence for as long as possible; (2) access to reliable information regarding what the future might hold; and (3) provision of a coordinated package of care with a single point of contact, usually a Clinical Nurse Practitioner.

Our patient was prescribed L-DOPA with carbidopa (co-careldopa, sinimet). Three months later he had noticed a substantial improvement in his tremor and his walking on 600 mg of L-DOPA per day in divided doses. However, some problems with unsteadyiness remained.

The response to L-DOPA therapy is very supportive of a diagnosis of idiopathic PD. While further increases in his L-DOPA dose might improve things slightly, most patients find that some symptoms do remain despite optimisation of their drug treatment. It is likely that over time his response to treatment will decline despite increasing doses of L-DOPA, and under those circumstances therapeutic manoeuvres include:

• Changing the interval between drug doses
• Prolonging the action of L-DOPA using sustained-release preparations or inhibitors of the enzymes responsible for dopamine breakdown MAO (e.g. selegiline) and COMT (e.g. entacapone)
• Providing the continuous delivery of short-acting dopamine agonists either subcutaneously (apomorphine) or transdermally (rotigotine).

Functional neurosurgery with implantation of electrodes for deep brain stimulation may have a role in the management of severe tremor or of L-DOPA-induced dyskinesias, but while some patients appear to derive substantial benefit, the results of randomised controlled trials are awaited.

CASE REVIEW

This late-middle-aged man presents with a very gradual onset of difficulty with walking. He also has a weak voice, difficulty using his hands, a tremor and is generally slowed up. With appropriate treatment there was substantial improvement in some of his symptoms, but he was by no means back to normal. It is likely that over time his symptoms will progress despite escalating treatments.

KEY POINTS

• While a pill-rolling tremor is often seen in patients with Parkinson's disease, it may not be what brings them to the doctor
• The symptoms of Parkinson's disease have often been present for years before medical attention is sought
• Therapies can go some way to replacing the dopaminergic deficit, but they neither reverse or halt the underlying neurodegenerative process
• Problems with unsteadiness are often much more resistant to treatment than, for instance, tremor

Further reading and references

Clarke CE. Clinical review: Parkinson's disease. *BMJ* 2007;**335**: 441–5.

A 49-year-old man with burning in the feet and difficulty walking

PART 2: CASES

Colin Flannigan is a 49-year-old plasterer who is referred to the outpatient clinic with symptoms of pain in his feet and difficulty in walking. On more detailed questioning he has noticed 'numbness' over the soles of his feet for the past 10 months. He has been troubled by a 'pins and needles' sensation and, more recently, 'burning' pains in both his feet as if they are 'on fire'. He also reports that his legs seem 'heavier', as if he is 'walking with concrete blocks on' and that he has become increasingly unsteady such that he has recently given up work. In particular he has noticed difficulties walking down stairs and he frequently catches his feet on rugs, curbs and steps.

Where might the anatomical site of his problem be (muscle, nerve, spinal cord, brainstem or cerebral hemispheres)?

The symptoms of numbness, pins and needles and burning indicate *paraesthesia*. The 'heaviness' and difficulties with walking suggest associated weakness of the legs. Both symptoms may arise due to a disorder affecting the peripheral nerves. Sensory symptoms and unsteadiness may also occur as a result of sensory pathways being affected by pathology affecting dorsal columns in the spinal cord. Unsteadiness may also arise as a consequence of disorders affecting the cerebellar system, and weakness and unsteadiness may arise in disorders affecting the spinocerebellar tracts.

Further history reveals that Mr Flannigan takes no regular prescribed medications although has been purchasing increasing quantities of painkillers from the supermarket for symptom relief. He has smoked 20 cigarettes a day for the past 35 years and admits to spending more time in the pub since giving up work.

Neurology: Clinical Cases Uncovered, 1st edition. © M. Macleod, M. Simpson and S. Pal. Published 2011 by Blackwell Publishing Ltd.

Examination reveals symmetrical distal sensory loss to light touch and pin prick in the lower limbs in addition to distal atrophy and weakness. Knee and ankle reflexes are absent even with reinforcement. There is no significant postural drop in his blood pressure.

What do the examination findings point to in terms of where in the nervous system the problem lies?

The examination findings reveal a 'stocking' distribution of sensory loss with muscle wasting and weakness distally. Together with the absence of reflexes, these findings point to a lower motor neuron problem, specifically one affecting the peripheral nerves, resulting in a peripheral neuropathy.

How common are peripheral neuropathies and what is the most common cause of peripheral neuropathies in the Western world?

Peripheral neuropathy is a common neurological problem affecting 2400 per 100 000. It is especially prevalent in people over the age of 65 years, where at least 7% of the population have symptoms of peripheral neuropathy; many more have abnormal neurological signs, and up to 70% of the over 65s have absent ankle reflexes. In the West, the most common cause of peripheral neuropathy is diabetes mellitus. However, leprosy (*Mycobacterium leprae*) is the primary cause in areas such as Southeast Asia, India and Africa.

What symptoms may patients with peripheral neuropathy present with?

As in Mr Flannigan's case, patients may present clinically with altered sensation (paraesthesia and hypoaesthesia), pain, weakness and loss of reflexes. Involvement of the autonomic system may result in symptoms such as postural hypotension, impotence and disordered sweating.

What are the principal anatomical components that make up the peripheral nerve and how may pathology of these anatomical structures lead to disorders of the peripheral nerve?

Peripheral nerves consist of two main structures: the axon and the myelin sheath. The vaso nervorum provides the blood supply. In peripheral neuropathy the axons, surrounding myelin sheath and vaso nervorum are targets for pathology. There are six principal ways in which a peripheral nerve may be damaged:

1 Demyelination: a process by which Schwann cells are damaged leading to slower conduction velocities, e.g. Guillain–Barré syndrome.
2 Axonal degeneration, e.g. toxic neuropathies.
3 Wallerian degeneration: direct trauma, e.g. nerve section, with consequent degeneration of the axon and distal myelin sheath.
4 Compression: sustained mechanical force disrupts the myelin sheath causing focal demyelination in entrapment neuropathies, e.g. carpal tunnel syndrome.
5 Infarction: microinfarction of the vaso nervorum compromises blood supply to the nerve, e.g. diabetes and vasculitis.
6 Infilitration: peripheral nerves are damaged by inflammation in infection (e.g. leprosy), malignancy, granulomatous disease (e.g. sarcoidosis) or amyloidosis.

Neuropathies may be classfied as mononeuropathies or polyneuropathies.

Which mononeuropathies are you aware of?

Mononeuropathies comprise a focal lesion of a single peripheral nerve. They may arise as a result of trauma, compression or entrapment.

Peripheral nerve compression or entrapment is exemplified by carpal tunnel syndrome in which the median nerve is compressed at the wrist. Acute compression can affect nerves exposed anatomically, for example tight plaster casts may compress the common peroneal nerve at the fibula head or so-called Saturday night palsy (compression of the radial nerve against the humerus). Other nerves commonly affected include the ulnar nerve compression and compression of the lateral cutaneous nerve of the leg in meralgia paraesthetica.

Multifocal neuropathy occurs when several separate peripheral nerves are affected either simultaneously or sequentially. High on the list of causes of multifocal neuropathy is systemic vasculitis (polyarteritis nodosa, Churg–Strauss disease) or a connective tissue disorder (rheumatoid arthritis, Sjögren's syndrome). Other causes include diabetes mellitus, leprosy, sarcoidosis, amyloidosis, malignancy, neurofibromatosis, HIV infection, Guillain–Barré syndrome and idiopathic multifocal motor neuropathy.

What features of the presenting complaint in the history are important in determining the cause and type of neuropathy?

Determining the acuity, rate of progression and pattern of nerve disturbance can be helpful diagnostically. In addition to their pathological causes, peripheral neuropathies can also be classified as: acute or chronic, symmetrical or asymmetrical, and focal or multifocal.

What features in the past medical history may be relevant?

A number of general systemic illnesses can contribute to peripheral neuropathies so it is important to enquire about the patient's past medical history and current state of health. The commonest cause of a peripheral neuropathy in the United Kingdom is diabetes mellitus. Other causes include rheumatoid arthritis, malignancy, connective tissue diseases, hypothyroidism, pernicious anaemia, HIV and sarcoidosis.

Which drugs may cause a peripheral neuropathy?

Many drugs can cause a peripheral neuropathy so taking an accurate history of current medications, as well as over-the-counter drugs and a full past treatment history is crucial. Drugs such as amiodarone, metronidazole, cisplatin and vincristine are examples, although there are many others.

What features in the family history are relevant?

A number of hereditary motor and sensory neuropathies (HMSN or Charcot–Marie–Tooth syndrome) have been identified for which there is often a clear family history of sensory symptoms and pes cavus in other family members. A hereditary liability to pressure palsies is an inherited cause of recurrent focal neuropathy.

What is important in the social and occupational history?

It is important to ask about social habits that may predispose to neuropathies, in particular alcohol intake, recreational drugs and risk factors for HIV and other infectious diseases. Occupational exposure to certain toxins may also be relevant.

What investigations would you request for Mr Flannigan?

The goals of investigation are to establish a diagnosis of peripheral neuropathy, determining whether an axonal or demyelinating neuropathy is present, to exclude conditions that may cause similar symptoms, and, if possible, to establish the underlying cause.

Common neuropathies may often be diagnosed by following the history, examination findings and results of basic (stage 1) investigations:

1 Blood tests, including full blood count, fasting blood glucose, renal function, liver function, thyroid function, vitamin B12, folic acid, methylmalonic acid and homocysteine, ESR, CRP and serum protein electrophoresis.
2 Urinalysis including for glucose and protein electrophoresis with immunofixation.

Colin Flannigan's blood test results are shown in Box 16.1.

What are the main abnormalities?

He has a macrocytic anaemia with deranged liver function tests and a low vitamin B12 level.

Which common toxic, metabolic and vitamin deficiency neuropathies are you aware of?

Metabolic neuropathies

1 Diabetes mellitus causes varied patterns of disorder: symmetrical sensory polyneuropathy, acute painful neuropathy, mononeuroapthy and multiple mononeuropathy (cranial nerve lesions and isolated peripheral nerve lesions), diabetic amyotrophy (painful neuropathy affecting the lower limbs due to infarction in the microcirculation of the lumbar sacral plexus) and autonomic neuropathy.
2 Uraemia: in renal failure the chronic high levels of uraemia result in a progressive sensorimotor neuropathy.

Box 16.1 Colin Flannigan's blood tests	
Haemoglobin (Hb)	10.8 g/dl
White cell count (WCC)	5.4 × 10⁹/L
Haematocrit (Hct)	0.465
Mean corpuscular volume (MCV)	102.6 fl
Platelets	287 × 10⁹/L
Sodium	137 mmol/L
Potassium	4.4 mmol/L
Urea	4.1 mmol/L
Creatinine	71 µmol/L
Bilirubin	30 mmol/L
Alkaline transferase	92 U/L
Albumin	53 U/L
Alkaline phosphatase	54 U/L
Gamma-glutamyl transpeptidase	170 IU/L
Calcium	2.15 mmol/L
Thyroid-stimulating hormone	2.25 mU/L
Thyroxine (T4)	16.5 nmol/L
Vitamin B12	195 ng/L
Folate	10.9 µg/L
Random glucose	5.8 mmol/L
Fasting glucose	4.2 mmol/L
Erythrocyte sedimentation rate	8
C-reactive protein (CRP)	4
Serum protein electrophoresis	Normal
Rheumatoid factor	Negative

PART 2: CASES

3 Thyroid disease: both hyperthyroidism and hypothyroidism can result in a mild chronic sensorimotor neuropathy.
4 Porphyria produces a severe, proximal neuropathy.
5 Amyloidosis produces polyneuropathy or multifocal neuropathy.
6 Refsum's disease is an autosomal recessive disease due to defective phytanic acid metabolism (a component of chlorophyll) and subsequent accumulation, producing a sensorimotor polyneuropathy

Toxic neuropathies

1 Alcohol excess produces a painful polyneuropathy of the lower limbs. Thiamine does alleviate symptoms to a degree but only complete abstinence halts progression.
2 Drugs and industrial toxins may produce a polyneuropathy.
3 Lead poisoning motor neuropathy.
4 Arsenic and thallium produce a polyneuropathy that may initially be sensory.

Vitamin deficiency neuropathies

1 Thiamin (vitamin B1) deficiency produces poly-neuropathy and cardiac failure. The disease of deficiency is beri beri and Wernicke–Korsakoff psychosis may result.

2 Pyridoxine (vitamin B6) deficiency produces a sensory neuropathy.

3 Cobalamin (vitamin B12) deficiency results in damage to the spinal cord, peripheral nerves and brain.

What other tests may be useful in assessment of peripheral neuropathies?

Stage 2 investigations include:

1 Neurophysiological tests: these comprises two parts – an electrical nerve conduction study (NCS) and electro-myography (EMG) – and can determine whether the neuropathy is demyelinating (with reduction in conduction velocities) or axonal (resulting in decreased amplitude of responses).

2 Biochemistry: serum protein electrophoresis and serum angiotensin-converting enzyme.

3 Immunology: antinuclear factor, anti-extractable nuclear antigen antibodies (anti-Ro, anti-La) and antineutrophil cytoplasmic antigen antibodies.

4 Anti-HIV antibodies.

5 Molecular genetic tests for inherited neuropathies

What other tests may be relevant in investigation of peripheral neuropathies?

Other tests which may be useful in the diagnosis of peripheral neuropathy include:

1 CSF examination: especially in inflammatory demyelinating neuropathies to look for an elevated CSF protein level. Inflammatory neuropathies may also lead to an elevated CSF white cell count.

2 MRI/CT of the spine: for herniated discs, spinal stenosis and the exclusion of other diseases causing similar symptoms.

3 Nerve biopsy: this involves removing and examining a sample of nerve tissue, most often from the lower leg (sural nerve). A biopsy may provide additional information about the type and degree of nerve damage, but it is an invasive procedure that is difficult to perform and may itself cause neuropathic side effects.

4 Skin biopsy: a sample of skin is removed allowing nerve fibre endings to be examined.

Mr Flanningan's nerve conduction study results show the following:

1 Sural nerve sensory action potentials demonstrate a reduction in conduction velocity. Motor conduction studies of the tibial and peroneal nerves demonstrate slightly reduced conduction velocity.

2 Needle electromyography examination of the distal lower limb muscles shows active denervation as well as chronic changes in the form of re-innervation patterns.

More detailed questioning reveals that Mr Flannigan has been drinking excessively for several years. Over the past 3 months he has been drinking up to half a bottle of vodka and several pints of beer a day.

What is the most likely diagnosis in this case?

This case highlights alcoholic neuropathy. Sensory symptoms, which are usually distal and symmetrical, include early numbness, followed by dysaesthesias, particularly at night. Progression to severe pain that is described as burning or lancinating may occur. Motor manifestations include distal weakness and muscle wasting. Autonomic disturbances are less common than in other neuropathies. The diagnosis is based on accurate history of prolonged and excessive alcohol intake, clinical signs and symptoms, and electrophysiological testing.

How would you manage Mr Flannigan's case?

Management is directed at limiting degeneration of the peripheral nerves and promoting restoration of normal function primarily through abstinence from alcohol. Nutritional support via a balanced diet and vitamin B supplementation are adjuncts to therapy along with active rehabilitation.

Neuropathic pain may be treated with drugs such as gabapentin, carbamazepine and amitriptyline. A multi-disciplinary approach may be needed with involvement of occupational therapists and physiotherapists. Walking sticks, crutches and walking frames may all be useful. Other practical measures include use of chiropody, weight reduction, sensible shoes, supportive foot wear and ankle–foot orthoses.

What is Mr Flannigan's prognosis?

The prognosis of alcoholic neuropathy is generally good provided alcohol intake is discontinued and other causes of neuropathy (such as malignancy and diabetes) are carefully excluded. Clinical and electrophysiological examinations are reported to improve even in the elderly.

CASE REVIEW

Progressive, unpleasant, distal lower limb sensory symptoms with associated difficulties in walking raise the possibility of a peripheral neuropathy. Examination findings that support a diagnosis of a mixed motor and sensory peripheral neuropathy include distal weakness, absent reflexes and a stocking distribution of sensory loss. There are a number of causes of such a neuropathy including diabetes, nutritional deficiencies, alcohol excess, inflammatory neuropathies and inherited neuropathies. Simple blood tests and neurophysiological studies may assist in establishing the diagnosis. In the case of alcohol-related neuropathy, nutritional supplements and cessation of alcohol offer the best course of outcome.

KEY POINTS

- Peripheral neuropathy is a common cause of neurological symptoms
- Neuropathies can be classified as axonal or demyelinating, motor, sensory or mixed, symmetrical or asymmetrical, and focal or multifocal
- They can also be classified according to whether they are acute, subacute or chronic
- Diabetes is the commonest cause of peripheral neuropathy in the United Kingdom
- There are numerous other causes including alcohol excess, nutritional deficiencies, metabolic derangement, drugs and inherited neuropathies
- First-line investigations include simple blood tests to investigate for the common nutritional, endocrine and inflammatory causes
- Nerve conduction studies are useful in establishing whether a neuropathy is present and if it is an axonal or demyelinating neuropathy
- Medical management depends on the underlying cause but may include tight glycaemic control on diabetic neuropathy, supplementation of vitamins in nutritional deficiency, cessation of drugs and alcohol in toxic neuropathies and treatment with immunomodulatory drugs in inflammatory neuropathies
- Patients may benefit from physiotherapy and occupational therapy input

PART 2: CASES

Further reading and references

England JD, Asbury AK. Seminar. Peripheral neuropathy. *Lancet* 2004;**363**:2151–61.

Hughes RAC. Clinical review. Regular review: peripheral neuropathy. *BMJ* 2002;**324**:466–9.

Case 17 A 72-year-old woman with memory problems

Audrey Brown is a 72-year-old retired occupational health nurse. She attends clinic with her husband. As far as Mrs Brown is concerned, she has no complaints and does not understand why she has been sent an appointment for a medical review. The referral letter from her GP reports that she has been experiencing difficulties with forgetfulness.

How would you proceed with this consultation?

Patients with cognitive difficulties frequently have little or no insight into their symptoms. Consultations need to be conducted with patience and empathy and a collateral history from a next of kin or carer is crucial. Ideally, this is gained in the presence of the patient but if necessary additional history may need to be sought over the telephone or in writing.

Jack Brown, Audrey's husband has also attended the clinic. He reports that she 'hasn't been right' for some time. The first sign something was wrong came about when the couple were on holiday in Spain 2 years ago and Audrey got lost in the hotel. This came as a surprise as they have stayed in the same hotel a number of times over the past few years. Since then, Mrs Brown has been increasingly forgetful, missing routine appointments and seemingly experiencing difficulties remembering contents of recent conversations. She no longer seems to enjoy hobbies such as gardening and reading and is unable to follow a television programme from start to finish. Over the past year, Mr Brown has had to take over doing all of the shopping and cooking and also manages all the household accounts.

What other questions in the history are important to ask in terms of establishing a diagnosis?

There are a number of features to consider when taking a history from a patient presenting with cognitive symptoms, including:

1 Have symptoms emerged and then progressed gradually, in a stepwise fashion, or with relentless deterioration?
2 Does the patient have vascular risk factors?
3 Is there a family history of cognitive or psychiatric impairment?
4 Is there a personal or family history of alcohol excess?
5 Has the patient been experiencing visual or auditory hallucinations?
6 Has there been a change in personality? For example, is the patient more withdrawn, emotionally labile, gregarious, inappropriate, obsessive, compulsive?
7 Are there symptoms of depression?

Mr Brown reports that his wife's symptoms have progressed gradually. Although he finds it difficult to gauge a change from day to day, their daughter who visits once a month confirms there has been a steady but definite deterioration. More recently her family have noticed that she struggles with tasks such as cooking meals and operating her television remote control. There are no symptoms of hallucinations. Although Mrs Brown is less interested in previous hobbies, her mood seems positive and she is not inappropriately tearful or happy. Her past medical history includes hypertension for which she takes bendroflumethazide. There is no family history of cognitive impairment in her parents or siblings and she drinks alcohol only very occasionally.

Neurology: Clinical Cases Uncovered, 1st edition. © M. Macleod, M. Simpson and S. Pal. Published 2011 by Blackwell Publishing Ltd.

Box 17.1 Summary of Alzheimer's disease (AD)

- AD is the commonest type of dementia and is characterised by the presence of memory problems associated with difficulties with language, praxis, agnosia and executive function
- Memory loss tends to be insidious with gradual progression
- 20–40% of patients experience delusions and hallucinations
- 25% of patients have symptoms of depression
- Extrapyramidal symptoms emerge in up to 60% (rigidity, bradykinesia, postural instability)
- Seizures occur in 10–20%
- There is a significant impact on daily social and work function

Box 17.2 Summary of vascular dementia

- Patients may have a history of previous strokes, transient ischaemic attacks, ischaemic heart disease, hypertension and hypercholesterolaemia
- Symptoms depend on the location of ischaemic events and include cognitive slowing, memory impairment and emotional lability
- The disease course is characterised by a stepwise rather than progressive worsening of symptoms as new ischaemic events occur
- Aphasia, apraxia and visuospatial impairments are seen in patients with cortical infarcs
- Gait abnormalities may be present

Box 17.3 Summary of dementia with Lewy bodies

Patients have memory problems with:

- Fluctuations in cognitive impairment
- Visual hallucinations
- Extrapyramidal (Parkinsonian) motor features

Box 17.4 Rarer causes of dementia

- Hypothyroidism
- Syphilis
- Chronic renal or hepatic failure
- HIV dementia
- Multiple sclerosis
- Huntington's disease
- Wilson's disease
- Corticobasal degeneration
- Prion diseases including Creutzfeldt–Jakob disease

17.4). With an aging population, dementia is increasingly contributing a significant medical and social burden. The prevalence doubles every 5 years after the age of 65 (prevalence 2% aged 65 years, 35% aged 85 years).

What general medical problems should be considered when assessing a patient with dementia?

Endocrine, infective and metabolic causes of cognitive impairment are potentially reversible and should be examined and investigated for. Conditions to consider include hypothyroidism, pernicious anaemia, syphilis, HIV, chronic liver and renal disease.

What specific bedside cognitive tests could be employed in assessing Mrs Brown?

The most commonly used bedside cognitive tests include the Abbreviated Mental Test Score, the Mini-Mental State Examination (MMSE) and the Addenbrooke's Cognitive Examination (ACE). However, the widespread use of some of these tools is limited by copyright protection.

Mrs Brown scores 22/30 on the MMSE dropping 3 points for orientation, 1 point for attention and calculation, 3 points for delayed recall of three objects, and 1 point for copying a figure of intersecting pentagons. Her general systemic

What are the common causes of memory impairment that should be considered in this case?

Mrs Brown has dementia. This is defined as 'problems with memory associated with deficits in other cognitive domains such as language, motor function, perception and executive functioning (which includes insight, planning or problem solving)'. Symptoms ultimately impact on daily functioning, resulting in interference with work and social activities. The common causes in the United Kingdom in order of frequency are Alzheimer's disease (50%; Box 17.1), vascular dementia (25%; Box 17.2), dementia with Lewy bodies (15%; Box 17.3) and frontotemporal dementia. Rarer dementia syndromes should also be considered as many of these are treatable (Box

examination, including blood pressure, is unremarkable. Apart from her cognitive problems, the remainder of her neurological examination is also unremarkable with no evidence of extrapyramidal signs, involuntary movements or ataxia.

Blood tests include a normal full blood count, erythrocyte sedimentation rate (ESR), electrolytes, serum B12, thyroid function tests, syphilis serology and antinuclear antibody. An MRI scan of the brain demonstrated hippocampal atrophy, consistent with Alzheimer's disease. An electroencephalogram demonstrated generalised slowing. A CSF examination performed to exclude infective or inflammatory causes for Mrs Brown's symptoms demonstrated a normal cell count and protein with no oligoclonal bands present.

What is the most likely diagnosis in this case?

The pattern of symptoms, nature of their onset and progression, and selective hippocampal atrophy on neuroimaging are consistent with a diagnosis of Alzheimer's disease (AD).

Which genes have been implicated in familial Alzheimer's disease?

The majority of cases of AD are 'sporadic'. However, approximately 15% of cases of AD are familial with an autosomal dominant pattern of inheritance. Three genes have been identified, β-amyloid precursor protein (APP, chromosome 21), presenilin 1 (PSEN-1, chromosome 14) and presenilin 2 (PSEN-2, chromosome 1), mutations of which lead to an AD-like phenotype, usually with an earlier age of onset than is typical for 'sporadic' AD. These genes are currently not tested in routine clinical practice but may be considered in patients with a strong family history or unusually early age of onset in the context of a research project.

How would you manage Mrs Brown at this point?

The management involves a multidisciplinary approach focusing on the psychosocial impact of the disease on the patient and care givers, nursing issues and drug treatment of individual symptoms. Patients, family and carers should be educated regarding the nature of underlying dementia and the support services available. Patients vary in terms of their insight and ability to retain information. Patients often benefit from following a routine with familiar loved ones and carers. A care plan should be established to target troublesome symptoms that may

emerge, including wandering, aggression, disinhibition, disrupted sleep, disturbed appetite and depression. Symptoms may progress over years and the mean time from diagnosis to death is 8 years. In the terminal state of illness, patients may be bed bound and mute with limb contractures and myoclonus. Death usually occurs secondary to infections of the chest or urine.

Mrs Brown's family was given contact details of the Alzheimer's Disease Association. Following liaison with social services, her GP arranged for access to a local day centre. In addition, a carer spends time with Mrs Brown once a week, allowing Mr Brown time to pursue activities out of the house. Mr Brown gained advice from his solicitor and was granted power of attorney for his wife.

Mrs Brown's family is keen to know if there are any tablets that she may take to improve her symptoms. What is the role of drug treatment in Alzheimer's disease?

There are currently no curative treatments for Alzheimer's disease. A careful trial of a cholinesterase inhibitor such as donepezil, rivastigmine or galantamine may contribute to a transient benefit in patients with mild to moderately severe disease. In reality, many patients experience little symptomatic benefit and may experience adverse side effects. Other drugs such as benzodiazepenes, antipsychotics and antidepressants are directed at modifying undesirable or dangerous behaviour but may in turn result in adverse side effects.

CASE REVIEW

Alzheimer's disease is the commonest form of dementia, usually seen in advanced years and characterised by memory impairment, personality change and language dysfunction. Patients may lack insight into their symptoms and need to be shown dignity, patience and respect. A careful collateral history needs to be gained from a family member or care giver. Bedside cognitive tests such as the MMSE and ACE-R are useful tools for assessing patients with dementia. Characteristic patterns of atrophy may also be seen on MRI of the brain. Management of patients with AD is multidisciplinary and patient-focused. Unnecessary drugs should be avoided and cholinesterase inhibitors considered in a well-selected subgroup. Family members and carers must be supported through the illness of their loved one.

KEY POINTS

- Dementia is becoming increasingly common with an aging population
- The commonest causes are Alzheimer's disease, vascular dementia, dementia with Lewy bodies and frontotemporal dementia
- The history is crucial in establishing diagnosis and detailed collateral accounts of symptom progression need to be gathered from those close to the patient
- Investigation of patients must include those targeted at rarer but reversible causes of dementia
- There are no curative treatments for the commonest dementias and multidisciplinary management is symptomatic, patient-focused and must take into account the burden placed on loved ones as carers

Further reading and references

Burns A, Iliffe S. Clinical review: dementia. *BMJ* 2009;**338**:b75.

Case 18 A 54-year-old woman with tingling hands

Mrs Berry, a 54-year-old kitchen assistant, complained to her general practitioner of gradually increasing discomfort in her hands and forearms which was interfering with her work.

What are the key features of the history?

1 What is the duration and the progression of her symptoms?

2 Are the hands affected equally, and is she right- or left-handed?

3 Is there any associated weakness?

4 What is its character of the discomfort?

- How severe is it?
- What is its distribution
- Is it provoked by neck movement
- Is it provoked by wrist position (driving, reading newspaper, sleeping)
- Can she do anything to relieve her discomfort

5 Does she have any relevant associated medical history?

- Diabetes
- Hypothyroidism
- Osteoarthritis
- Acromegaly
- Pregnancy
- Neck trauma

The discomfort began some 9 months ago and was initially restricted to her right hand; she is right-handed. Since then, things have become gradually and inexorably worse such that her left hand is also affected, and the discomfort extends proximally almost to her elbow on the right. She describes a tingling numbness over the thumb and first two fingers, and reports that this is worse at night (when it can

wake her from sleep), and that during the daytime it can be precipitated by reading the newspaper, talking on the telephone for too long and by driving. There is no associated medical history except for a mild whiplash injury sustained some 20 years previously.

What is the likely differential diagnosis?

The first question relates to the location of the lesion. Given the bilateral, asymmetrical and progressive onset, a single central lesion (brain or spinal cord) is improbable, and a peripheral lesion (nerve root, peripheral nerve) is more likely. If this is due to a peripheral lesion, it must be multifocal (because no one nerve supplies both hands). Because the legs are not affected it is unlikely to be due to a generalised problem with nerve function, and is more likely to be due to localised problems such as compression of nerves or nerve roots.

In her case, there are a number of features that suggest that the problem may be due to compression of the median nerve in the carpal tunnel, or carpal tunnel syndrome. These are:

1 She works with her hands: carpal tunnel syndrome is very much more common in those who work with their hands, and can be considered to be an occupational disease.

2 Her dominant right hand was affected first.

3 The distribution of the most intense sensory disturbance is that of the median nerve.

4 The discomfort wakes her from sleep.

5 Her symptoms are provoked by activities that lead to wrist flexion.

With this sensory distribution, the differential diagnosis is of bilateral compression of the C6 nerve root in the neck, most likely due to a cervical spondylitic radiculopathy. The extension of pain and sensory symptoms proximal to the wrist is commonly reported by patients with carpal tunnel syndrome.

Neurology: Clinical Cases Uncovered, 1st edition. © M. Macleod, M. Simpson and S. Pal. Published 2011 by Blackwell Publishing Ltd.

Establishing the diagnosis: examination

If her symptoms are indeed due to carpal tunnel syndrome then we would expect to find evidence of median nerve motor and sensory dysfunction in the hand. Alternatively, if her symptoms are due to a cervical spondylitic radiculopathy (nerve root dysfunction), we would expect evidence of a C6 radiculopathy and, possibly, of an associated myelopathy (spinal cord dysfunction).

On inspection of the hands she has some loss of muscle bulk at the base of the thumb (the thenar eminence) on the right, and to a lesser extent on the left hand. In the right hand there is weakness of opposition (opponens pollicis) and abduction (abductor pollicis brevis) of the thumb, but abduction of the index finger and the bulk of the first dorsal interosseous muscle are normal. Similar but less marked findings are observed in the left hand. In the sensory examination there is reduced sensation to light touch and to pin prick over the right thumb, index and middle finger and contiguous palm and over the left thumb and index finger. When she is asked to hyperextend her wrists (placing the palms of her hands together as if praying, and bringing the hands down such that her forearms form a straight line), her typical symptoms begin within about 15 seconds, and are relieved within a minute or so of changing position.

What is the likely diagnosis?

The history and examination are typical of carpal tunnel syndrome, where the median nerve is compressed within the wrist between the carpal bones posteriorly and the transverse carpal ligament anteriorly. Bending the wrist reduces the transverse diameter of the carpal tunnel (imagine bending the inside of a kitchen roll holder) leading to compression of the median nerve and its dysfunction. Clinical features helping to distinguish between carpal tunnel syndrome (CTS) and a C6 radiculopathy are given in Table 18.1.

How might the diagnosis be confirmed?

The diagnosis can be confirmed by electrophysiological evidence of median nerve dysfunction localised within the carpal tunnel. The purpose of such testing is not to document median nerve dysfunction (the sensitivity of nerve conduction studies (NCS) in the diagnosis of CTS is less than 80%, and in patients being considered for surgery it has a negative predictive value – correctly predicting that patients with normal NCS will not benefit from surgery – of only 14%), but rather to demonstrate the absence of other conditions such as a more wide-

Table 18.1 Discrimination between carpal tunnel syndrome (CTS) and C6 radiculopathy.

	CTS	C6 radiculopathy
Pain	Wrist and hand, occasionally forearm; usually beginning in the dominant hand	
Timing	At night, wakes from sleep	On movement, lifting
Relieving factors	Patient demonstrated shaking wrist	Lateral arm, dorsal forearm
Provocation	Tinel's sign (percussion over wrist); Phalen's sign (wrist flexion to 90° for 30 seconds)	
Sensory findings	Lateral two-thirds of the palm, lateral three and a half fingers; sensation on thenar eminence spared	Lateral forearm, first and second digits
Motor findings	Abductor pollicis brevis, opponens pollicis	Forearm flexion, pronation, wrist and finger extension
Reflex change	None	Biceps, brachioradialis

spread subclinical neuropathy which might predispose the median nerve to involvement and which might limit the therapeutic response to surgery.

Nerve conduction studies in the arms show normal distal motor latencies in the ulnar nerve bilaterally, with delayed motor latencies in the median nerve more marked in the right than the left side. Median nerve sensory action potentials are of reduced amplitude and of increased latency.

These neurophysiological findings are typical of carpal tunnel syndrome, without evidence of an accompanying peripheral neuropathy.

How should patients with carpal tunnel syndrome be managed?
Non-medical treatments

Where pain is the predominant symptom and where this is largely situational – i.e. occurring during specific tasks, or occurring predominantly at night – the use of a wrist splint to limit flexion and extension can lead to a marked reduction in symptoms. For some patients, this will be preferred to surgery (see below), and in all cases is a simple measure that can relieve symptoms while they wait for further investigation and for surgery.

Medical treatments

If there is inflammation in the wrist, inflammatory soft tissue within the carpal tunnel can contribute to the crowding that leads to pressure on the median nerve. Because of this, anti-inflammatory drugs may be of help. The two approaches are either of non-steroidal anti-inflammatory drugs (NSAIDs) such as ibuprofen or diclofenac, or corticosteroids given orally or by local injections. Meta-analysis of randomised controlled trials suggests that NSAIDs have limited efficacy and that the local injection of steroids is more effective than systemic steroids.

Surgery

Surgical decompression of the carpal tunnel is a straight-forward procedure, where the anterior carpal ligament is transsected, thereby increasing the cross-sectional area of the carpal tunnel and relieving the pressure on the median nerve. Meta-analysis of randomised controlled trials suggests that patients undergoing surgery have more than twice the chance of being free of symptoms at 1 year compared with those treated with wrist splints. Limited data from trials comparing surgery with steroid treatment suggest that both are effective in the short term, but that the benefits of surgery last longer.

She was referred to the local orthopaedic surgeons who carried out sequential carpal tunnel release procedures, and when seen for review 6 months later she reported substantial relief of her symptoms.

CASE REVIEW

This middle-aged woman with a manual occupation developed discomfort, initially in her dominant right hand. This was worse at night and on wrist extension, and is typical of carpal tunnel syndrome. The abnormal findings on examination suggested severe established disease, and she underwent surgery to good effect.

KEY POINTS

- Carpal tunnel syndrome is so common that people – presumably graphic artists with occupational CTS – draw cartoons about it
- The history is often typical (as here), and if examination is normal then initial treatment (e.g. wrist splints) can be introduced without waiting for nerve conduction studies to confirm the diagnosis
- CTS is more common in those who work with their hands, and it usually begins in the dominant hand
- The symptoms may extend proximally far beyond the wrist

Further reading and references

Verdugo RJ, Salinas RS, Castillo J, Cea JG. Surgical versus non-surgical treatment for carpal tunnel syndrome. *Cochrane Database Syst Rev* 2008;Issue 4:CD001552.

Case 19 A 26-year-old woman with right-sided weakness

Ellen Jacobs, a 26-year-old lawyer, is referred by her GP with a short history of right-sided weakness.

What are the key features of the history?
1 When did her symptoms begin?
2 How long did they take to reach their maximum severity, or are they still getting worse?
3 What is the distribution of the weakness?
4 How severe is the weakness? What does it prevent her from doing?
5 Has she had any previous episodes of neurological disturbance?
6 What are the associated symptoms?
   • Headache
   • Speech disturbance
   • Numbness or sensory loss
   • Visual loss
   • Disturbance of bladder or bowel function
   • Seizures, focal or generalised
7 Is there a family history?
8 Have there been any particularly stressful recent life events, and is there a history of medically unexplained symptoms such as fibromyalgia, irritable bowel syndrome or chronic fatigue syndrome?

She first became aware of a heaviness affecting her right hand and arm at the end of a busy day at work some 4 weeks ago, and thought she was simply tired. However, over the next few days the heaviness became a weakness and progressed to involve the whole arm. About a week after the onset of her symptoms in the hand she started to develop a heaviness in her right leg and a sensation that her leg was dragging while she walked. These symptoms had all progressed over the following 2 weeks, but over the last week had remained constant.

Neurology: Clinical Cases Uncovered, 1st edition. © M. Macleod, M. Simpson and S. Pal. Published 2011 by Blackwell Publishing Ltd.

At the time of her assessment her weakness involved the right arm and leg but not her face. She reported that she was still able to walk with the help of a stick, but found this to be very tiring and she had not been at work for the last fortnight. In addition to her weakness she reported that she had a tingling numbness of the right arm and leg as if she had been sleeping on it, but more intense, intrusive and at times almost painful. She reported no problems with speech or swallowing, coordination or bladder or bowel function and she had not had a headache at any stage. There is no family history of neurological disturbance, no recent life events, and her only past history is of a brief episode of depression some 5 years ago.

What is the likely differential diagnosis?
Her symptoms are most in keeping with a left hemisphere lesion involving the corticospinal tract. The differential diagnosis includes stroke, demyelination, migraine, a space-occupying lesion or a functional neurological problem. The lack of headache at any stage makes this unlikely to be migraine, and the pace of onset (slow rather than abrupt) is against stroke as a cause. Furthermore, the lack of speech disturbance is somewhat against a cortical lesion. Taken together, the features are most in keeping with demyelination, a space-occupying lesion or a functional neurological problem. The lack of antecedent stressful life events or medically unexplained symptoms is somewhat against a functional neurological problem, and while the occurrence of focal seizures in the right arm would argue strongly in favour of a space-occupying lesion such as a glioma, the absence of this in no way rules this out.

What are the key features of the examination?
In cases such as this the role of the examination is to confirm that the symptoms described are matched by signs of neurological impairment; to localise the lesion within the nervous system; and to seek evidence of other

neurological impairments that might reflect previous episodes of CNS demyelination in other parts of the nervous system.

Lesions in the corticospinal tract create an upper motor neuron or pyramidal weakness which is more apparent in the extensors of the arms and the flexors of the legs. Usefully, eversion of the forefoot is often markedly weaker than inversion. This pattern of weakness is associated with increased tone (due to autonomous and desuppressed activity of the spinal reflex arcs due to loss of descending inhibitory signalling), brisk reflexes and, in the legs, sustained clonus at the ankle and extensor plantar responses. There may be sensory changes due to involvement of adjacent spinothalamic and thalamocortical tracts, but while sensory extinction may be seen both with peripheral nerve and root and with cortical lesions, lesions in central pathways are more likely to result in altered perception of touch, and specifically a pins and needles type dysaesthesia in response to pin prick stimulation.

Although there is no history of speech disturbance, it is important to establish whether there are any subtle problems with comprehension or expressed speech that might indicate a cortically based lesion. Similarly, testing for a homonymous hemianopia or visuospatial neglect should be performed. The corticospinal tract may be involved as it passes through the brainstem, in which case there may be associated abnormalities of the cranial nerves or of cerebellar function.

A previous episode of optic neuritis may have left residual signs including disc pallor, optic atrophy, a relative afferent papillary deficit and/or reduced perception of colour in the affected eye.

Your patient had a pyramidal weakness affecting the right arm (flexors 4/5, extensors 4–/5) and leg (flexors 4/5, extensors 4+/5) with increased tone, brisk reflexes and an extensor plantar response on that side. She was aware of sensory stimulation throughout the right side, but felt pin prick and light touch as an unpleasant burning sensation. There were no abnormalities of speech, of the cranial nerves or of cerebellar function.

These findings are consistent either with a first episode of demyelination or with a left hemisphere space-occupying lesion such as a glioma. The tempo of onset of her symptoms, the relative incidence of demyelination and glioma in women of her age, and the observation that things are no longer getting worse all make demyelination substantially more likely than glioma.

What investigations are indicated at this stage?

She should have routine baseline blood tests taken, including an ESR and CRP, and she should also be tested for some of the systemic inflammatory disorders that can cause CNS demyelination (antinuclear factor, lupus anticoagulant). Urgent brain imaging is required to exclude a space-occupying lesion; ideally this would be MRI scanning as this might also show the characteristic features of demyelination. However, if urgent MRI is not available she should have CT scanning now pending later MRI.

All blood tests are normal. An MRI scan shows four areas of high signal on T2-weighted imaging, with lesions distributed around the ventricles (Fig. 19.1) and in the brainstem.

These findings are typical of demyelination such as is seen in multiple sclerosis (MS). However, as far as we know this is her first clinical episode, and so this is a clinically isolated syndrome rather than MS.

What causes demyelination?

The causes of demyelination are not known, but the pathophysiology is thought to involve autoimmunity directed against the myelin-bearing cells of the central nervous system (the oligodendrocyte). While in most cases this appears to be a cell-mediated autoimmunity, some closely related conditions (e.g. neuromyelitis optica) appear to be due to antibody-mediated autoimmunity (anti-aquaporin antibodies). The stimulus to autoimmunity is not known, but there are clearly both genetic and environmental factors, these latter perhaps including latitude (and/or sunlight exposure) and exposure to cytomegalovirus during a critical early period.

What is the risk of her going on to develop MS?

Eighty per cent of patients with a first episode of demyelination will go on to make a rapid and full recovery. However, over a 10-year period as many as three-quarters of patients may have a further clinical episode of demyelination and therefore develop MS. This risk is lower in patients with a normal MRI at presentation (around 80% of whom do not develop MS) and is higher, with more severe disease, the more lesions present on the MRI. Within 10 years, one-third of patients with 10 lesions or more on their presentation MRI are unable to walk 100 m without assistance. The risk can be further stratified by

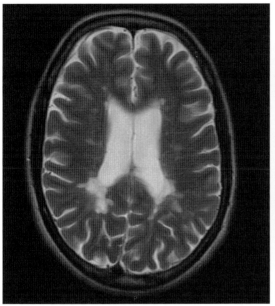
(a)

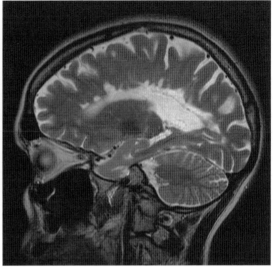
(b)

Figure 19.1 MRI of the brain for this patient with MS. There are a large number of mainly small, radially orientated lesions in relation to the periventricular white matter with thinning of the corpus callosum, which is also involved by these lesions. The lesions are rather more confluent around the posterior part of the lateral ventricle. There are some signal changes in the posterior pons just at the level of the middle cerebellar peduncles bilaterally and some minor signal changes in both the cerebellar hemispheres. The appearances are consistent with demyelination.

the presence of CSF oligoclonal bands (these are seen in around two-thirds of cinically isolated syndrome patients, but if they are not present the risk of developing MS over 6 years is only 16%).

How should patients with a clinically isolated syndrome be managed?

1 *Treatment of acute attack.* Early treatment with intravenous methylprednisolone may reduce the duration of symptoms, but does not appear to have any impact on either the extent of any residual disability or the risk of going on to develop MS. Even short courses of steroids are not without their side effects, so treatment is usually only given where there is clear disability and where symptoms are continuing to worsen.

2 *Modulation of the risk of developing MS.* There is now some evidence to suggest that initiation of MS 'disease-modifying therapies' after a first clinically isolated syndrome probably delays the progression to MS, but whether it actually prevents progression to MS in any patient is not clear. Given that many such patients would never develop MS anyway, the role of these treatments

for clinically isolated syndromes is not clear, and at present they are not routinely offered.

The potential risks and benefits of steroid treatment were discussed with the patient, and given that her symptoms were not interfering with her work, she decided not to go ahead with treatment. She was referred to the local MS specialist nurses who provided her with further information about the nature of clinically isolated syndromes and the potential treatments available. She was referred to the physiotherapist and occupational therapist. At review 8 weeks later she had made a full recovery. Having considered the risks and potential benefits of 'disease-modifying therapy' and the small amount of additional information that might be gained from repeat MRI scanning or lumbar puncture she elected not to proceed with further investigation or treatment, and she was discharged to the care of her GP.

Eighteen months later she developed, over the course of a week, problems with unsteadiness while walking, double vision and incoordination. Her GP telephoned the local MS nurses.

In all likelihood she is having a further episode of CNS inflammation. The priorities of care are to confirm the diagnosis, to support her through the diagnosis of MS, to initiate treatment with intravenous steroids if this is her wish, and to discuss again the issue of treatment with 'disease-modifying therapies'.

The MS nurses arrange for her to be seen by a neurologist the following day. On examination she has both truncal and limb ataxia, worse on the right; nystagmus in all directions of gaze; double vision at the extremes of lateral gaze with jumping vision; brisk reflexes; and bilaterally upgoing plantars. She elects to go ahead with i.v. steroids, and this is arranged on a day-patient basis. While she is receiving her treatment she meets with the MS nurses, who provide her with further information about the disease and the treatments available, and arrange for her to come back to discuss treatments with a consultant neurologist the following week.

What is the natural history of MS, and can this be modified by treatment?

When she comes back to the neurology clinic she is going to want to know what is likely to happen to her in the future, and whether any interventions can improve that prospect. Individual patients can be very different one from another, but it is possible to make some general statements. On average, patients with MS are about 1% more likely to die each year than patients without MS. The speed of disease progression is very variable, on average taking 10 years before patients experience sustained moderate disability and 24 years until patients need a stick to walk 100 m. Generally speaking, MS is more rapidly progressive in men, in older patients, in those with incomplete recovery from the first attack, and in those with frequent or early relapses. Systematic reviews of randomised controlled trials show that oral azathioprine, subcutaneous β-interferon or subcutaneous glatiramer acetate are effective in reducing the frequency of attacks and the accumulation of new lesions. There is little evidence to suggest that they have a substantial effect on the risk or extent of MS-related disability.

This is a field of rapid therapeutic development, most recently including immunosuppressive drugs such as mitoxantrone and natazulimab. Novel oral immunosuppressive drugs are in late development, but one of the frustrations of drug development in MS is the rather obvious constraint that long-term studies are required to show long-term benefits. Previous studies have shown that short-term improvements in relapse frequency or MRI appearances do not always translate into reductions in long-term disability, and the enthusiasm for novel therapeutics must be tempered, in discussion with patients, with an acknowledgment of our uncertainty about long-term risks and benefits.

CASE REVIEW

This woman presented with a subacute onset of right-sided weakness and numbness typical of demyelination. She elected not to have steroid treatment and went on to make a full recovery. However, 18 months later she presented with symptoms of brainstem dysfunction, and her conditional had evolved from a clinically isolated syndrome to multiple sclerosis.

KEY POINTS

- Inflammatory demyelinating lesions in the central nervous system are the most common cause of subacute neurological impairment in young adults
- A second episode – affecting a different part of the nervous system at a different time – is required for a diagnosis of MS
- Not everyone with demyelination goes on to get MS
- Not everyone with MS goes on to develop MS-related disability
- While treatments can reduce the severity (steroids) or frequency (azathioprine, interferon, glatiramer acetate) of relapses, they have little effect on the accumulation of MS-related disability

Further reading and references

Murray TJ. Clinical review. Diagnosis and treatment of multiple sclerosis. *BMJ* 2006;**332**:525–7.

A 19-year-old woman with acute headache and tingling

Monica is a 19-year-old student who presents to the accident and emergency department with headache. It is severe, and associated with nausea. Shortly before it came on she noticed a tingling sensation in her right arm and the right side of her face. She is worried she is having a stroke.

What are the key features of the history?

1 What is the duration of the headache?

2 Has she ever had one before?

3 How long did it take to reach its maximum severity?

4 What is the site of the headache? Unilateral or bilateral?

5 What is its character? Dull, throbbing, aching or sharp?

6 How severe is it? (mark out of 10)

7 What are the associated symptoms?
- Visual symptoms: jagged lines, flashing lights
- Speech disturbance
- Focal limb weakness or sensory symptoms
- Nausea or vomiting
- Photophobia (dislike of light)
- Phonophobia (dislike of noise)
- Fever

8 What are the possible triggers of this episode?
- Altered sleep pattern
- Missed meals
- Stress or relaxation after stress
- Foods and alcohol (particularly chocolate, cheese, wine)
- Drugs, e.g. glyceryl trinitrate, oral contraceptive pill
- Menstruation

9 Is there a family history of headaches or migraine?

The headache developed the previous day after her end-of-year history exam, and came on gradually, reaching

Neurology: Clinical Cases Uncovered, 1st edition. © M. Macleod, M. Simpson and S. Pal. Published 2011 by Blackwell Publishing Ltd.

its maximum severity over the course of about an hour. It is localised to the left side of her head, and is concentrated around the eye area. It is throbbing in nature, 6/10 severity and associated with nausea but she has not vomited. It is also associated with pins and needles in her right arm and the right side of her face, which spread gradually over a period of 10 minutes. Her speech and vision are not affected. Since it started, she has wanted to lie down in her bedroom with the lights off, and when she hears her room-mates playing loud music it makes the headache worse. Her mother and aunt suffered from headaches and regularly missed work because of this. She is afebrile and her blood pressure is normal. Full neurological examination, including fundoscopy, reveals no abnormalities.

What is the likely differential diagnosis?

The differential diagnosis is between a *primary* headache (e.g. migraine, tension-type headache, cluster headache) and headache which is *secondary* to another cause (e.g. subarachnoid haemorrhage, brain tumour, meningitis, giant cell arteritis). As a general rule, the length of the history is the most important factor in determining the likelihood of secondary headache and the need for further investigation. Short histories of sudden-onset headache need urgent investigation ± treatment; headaches lasting several months with no other symptoms are much less likely to be serious or life-threatening, although they may be highly disabling.

In this case, the history is typical for migraine with aura (Box 20.1), and in a patient of this age this is by far the most likely diagnosis. The headache is unilateral, throbbing and of moderate severity. Its onset was gradual over an hour, and it is associated with nausea, photophobia and phonophobia. It is preceded by focal sensory symptoms of the face and arm (an aura). Aura can take the form of any focal cerebral dysfunction, but most commonly involves flashing lights or jagged lines in one half of the visual field. In her case, the probable trigger is relaxation after the stress of her exam. There is a positive

> **Box 20.1 Abridged version of International Headache Society criteria for migraine**
>
> **Migraine without aura**
> Headache lasting 4 hours to 3 days
> Nausea/vomiting and/or light and noise sensitivity
> Two of the following:
> - Unilateral pain
> - Moderate or severe intensity pain
> - Aggravation by simple physical activity
> - Pulsating pain
>
> **Migraine with aura**
> At least three of the following:
> - Reversible brainstem or focal cortical dysfunction
> - Aura develops over >4 minutes, or two auras in succession
> - Each aura lasts <60 minutes
> - Headache of <60 minutes following an aura

> **Box 20.2 Acute treatments for migraine**
>
> - Aspirin 900–1200 mg orally. Soluble aspirin works more quickly and should be taken as close as possible to the onset of an attack
> - Paracetamol 1 g orally, again in soluble form
> - Domperidone 20 mg orally (or another prokinetic anti-emetic such as metaclopramide 10 mg orally) is useful, particularly where nausea is a prominent symptom
> - Triptans – these are a migraine-specific drug, whose effects are mediated via serotonin receptors ($5\text{-}HT_{1B}$). This specific receptor subtype is located on the cranial blood vessels, and agonists at this receptor (like the triptans) produce selective vasoconstriction in this area. If administered early in the attack, they are highly effective in aborting migrainous headache, but have no effect on aura or associated gastrointestinal symptoms

family history, which is often the case in migraine. However, the history is relatively short, and the differential diagnosis would include stroke and cerebral venous sinus thrombosis. It would be important to ask about a personal or family history of prothrombotic tendency, or the use of drugs such as the oral contraceptive pill which could increase the risk of stroke.

What causes migraine?

At one time the primary abnormality in migraine was believed to originate in the cerebral vasculature. However, more recent opinion holds that migraine occurs as a result of dysfunction of the neuronal networks responsible for pain, with either abnormal activation of the nociceptive pathways or failure of the inhibitory pathways which would normally suppress pain. The precise locus of the pathology is unknown, although studies using functional magnetic resonance imaging (fMRI) have suggested a source in the dorsolateral pons, possible in the noradrenergic neurons of the locus coeruleus. Changes in cerebral blood flow associated with migraine are believed to be a secondary phenomenon, rather than the root cause of the symptoms.

She returns for follow-up 3 months later. She is having three or four bouts of headache each month, and each one is lasting around 12 hours. She is missing university, and is worried she will have to resit the term.

How should patients with migraine be managed?
Lifestyle

Patients with migraine may benefit from lifestyle modifications, in order to reduce the frequency of attacks. These include:

1 Keeping regular hours, and avoiding sleep deprivation or oversleeping in the morning.
2 Eating regular meals (relative hypoglycaemia is thought to be a potent trigger).
3 Avoidance of dietary triggers, e.g. alcohol, chocolate, cheese.

Keeping a headache diary can be a useful way to identify lifestyle triggers and also to evaluate the efficacy of pharmaceutical therapies.

Drug treatment

Drug treatment for migraine (Box 20.2) can be categorised as acute rescue or prophylaxis.

Acute treatment
Acute rescue therapies should be used as soon as possible after the onset of an attack.

1 *Analgesia.* The first line of treatment is the use of standard analgesics such as aspirin, non-steroidal anti-

inflammatory drugs (ibuprofen, diclofenac) or paraceta-mol. These are more likely to be effective when given early in the course of an attack, so soluble preparations with rapid absorbtion are preferred. Where nausea or vomiting is a prominent feature of a patient's usual attack then domperidone or metcloplamide can also be given, again the earlier the better.

2 *Migraine-specific drugs: triptans.* There are several different triptans which have slightly different times of onset and durations of effect, and each is available in a number of formats. The choice of which particular triptan to use will be dictated by patient preference. For instance, some patients want the fastest possible onset of action, whereas others may prefer a longer lasting action. Some patients prefer oral medications, whereas in others nausea and vomiting may be prominent and subcutaneous administration is preferable. Triptans are very expensive, particularly the inhaled and parenteral forms. Furthermore, they are relatively contraindicated in patients with ischaemic heart disease (there are serotonergic receptors in the coronary circulation, and vasoconstriction here could exacerbate cardiac ischaemia). Side effects include chest pain (although studies have shown that this is only rarely associated with demonstrable cardiac ischaemia, and usually occurs in young patients with low cardiovascular risk factor profiles) and burning sensations in the face. They may also cause fatigue and dizziness. Triptans can also cause medication overuse headache (see Case 25) and it is essential that they are not used more than twice per week.

3 *Migraine-specific drugs: ergot derivatives.* These are another option for acute treatment; they also act on the serotonergic system causing vasoconstriction. They have similar side effects to the triptans but also cause muscle cramps and gastrointestinal upset, and they are also liable to overuse. Their side effects tend to be more frequent and more severe, hence they are seldom used in clinical practice unless other therapies have failed.

Prophylaxis

Prophylactic treatments (Table 20.1) can be used for patients who are having regular migraines that are disabling and interfering with their normal activities. In general, prophylaxis would not be considered for patients having fewer than two migraines per month (unless their headaches are very long-lasting or they are unable to

tolerate any acute treatments) although the threshold will vary between patients and the choice of agent will depend on co-morbid disease and side effect profile.

Monica's doctor educates her about the acute and prophylactic strategies for managing migraine, and encourages her to keep a diary to identify trigger factors. She discovers that her headaches are occurring almost exclusively on weekends when she sleeps in after a late night. However, she loves her lie-ins and doesn't want to miss out on the Friday night parties. She decides to start a prophylactic medication, amitryptiline, and the frequency of her migraines decreases markedly.

Table 20.1 Prophylactic treatment for migraine.

Drug	Mechanism	Side effects
Pizotifen	Serotonergic and histaminergic antagonist	Weight gain, drowsiness
Topiramate	Anticonvulsant	Weight loss, cognitive slowing, acute glaucoma, teratogenicity
Sodium valproate	Anticonvulsant	Hair loss, thrombocytopenia, hepatotoxicity, teratogenicity
Amitryptiline	Tricyclic antidepressant	Cardiac arrhythmias, antimuscarinic effects
Propranolol	Beta-blocker	Heart block, fatigue
Methysergide	Synthetic ergot alkaloid	Retroperitoneal fibrosis

CASE REVIEW

This patient presents with an acute headache with features of migraine (nausea, photophobia, throbbing headache, preceding aura). Clinical examination and brain imaging were normal and a diagnosis of migraine with aura was made. She went on to develop more frequent migraines and required a combination of acute treatments and prophylactic therapy, with good result.

KEY POINTS

- Migraine is a common primary headache and may or may not be associated with aura symptoms
- History-taking is vital in patients with headache
- The neurologist should always ask about migrainous features, such as:
  - unilateral headache
  - throbbing
  - photophobia/phonophobia
  - nausea
- Treatment for migraine can be divided into lifestyle measures, acute treatment and prophylaxis. In general, prophylaxis should be considered if patients are suffering more than 2 days a month

Further reading and references

Evers S, Afra J, Frese A, Goadsby P, Linde M, May A, Sandor P. EFNS guideline on the drug treatment of migraine – revised report of an EFNS task force. *Eur J Neurol* 2009;**16**:968–81.

James Patterson is a 63-year-old warehouseman who presents with a 3-month history of increasing difficulty at work. He feels generally weak, but complains that his hands in particular are becoming almost useless for manual tasks, and in fact he has been off work for the last month.

What are the key features of the history?

1 Is his weakness getting gradually worse, or has it been pretty fixed since the onset?
2 Is the weakness worse at any particular time of day, or does it seem to be exacerbated by exertion?
3 Is there any associated pain or cramp?
4 Is there associated disturbance of bowel or bladder function or of sensation?
5 What about other associations?
  • Weight loss
  • Skin rash
  • Difficulty with speech or swallowing
  • Dysarthria
  • Choking on food
  • Liquids escaping down the nose while drinking ('nasal escape')
  • Dry mouth
  • Double vision
  • Shortness of breath on exertion
  • Morning headache or excessive daytime sleepiness
6 Is there a family history?

The weakness has developed insidiously over 3 months, and he reports that his wife thinks it has been going on for substantially longer. He simply cannot function at work because he is losing grip in his hands. As far as he can tell

there is no pattern to his weakness, and he's not aware of anything that makes it better or worse.

The other important positive features in the history are that he has started to develop cramping pains in his legs at night, and has general muscle aches and pains; he finds it increasingly difficult to find a comfortable position in which to sleep. He has lost 12.5 kg in weight in the last 6 months, and while he has noticed no difficulties with eating he does report occasional nasal escape of fluids and his wife thinks his voice may have changed slightly.

On direct questioning he reports no disturbance of bladder or bowel function or of sensation, no double vision, skin rash or dryness of the mouth, and no fatiguable element to the weakness.

What is the likely differential diagnosis?

He describes an isolated problem with muscle power without associated sensory loss, fatiguability or systemic features apart from weight loss. The lack of sensory features makes a generalised sensorimotor neuropathy (such as Guillain–Barré syndrome) unlikely; in spite of the bulbar features (difficulty with talking and with swallowing), the lack of fatiguability makes myasthenia gravis unlikely; and the absence of a dry mouth makes the Lambert–Eaton myasthenic syndrome unlikely.

His problem seems to localise exclusively to the motor system, and the most likely diagnosis is of motor neuron disease. The differential diagnosis includes a primary problem with muscle (a myopathy), a mixed cervical and lumbar spondylitic radiculomyelopathy, multifocal motor neuropathy with conduction block, and Kennedy's disease. The examination should aim to help distinguish between these possibilities.

He walks into the consulting room with the aid of one stick, and as he introduces himself you note a marked dysarthria. On formal examination the upper cranial nerves are normal. He has a spastic, fasciculating and wasted tongue and a brisk jaw jerk. He has fasciculations in the

Neurology: Clinical Cases Uncovered, 1st edition. © M. Macleod, M. Simpson and S. Pal. Published 2011 by Blackwell Publishing Ltd.

small muscles of the hand, in the triceps bilaterally and in the supraspinatus and infraspinatus. There is no gynaecomastia. In the limbs he has pronounced wasting of the small muscles of the hand including the first dorsal interosseous bilaterally, with 4–/5 weakness in the hand muscles. Power proximally in the arms is 4+/5, reflexes are brisk and symmetrical and there are no abnormalities of sensation.

Similarly, in the legs he has fasciculation, weakness and wasting with normal sensation, brisk reflexes and bilaterally and symmetrically upgoing plantar responses.

What is the differential diagnosis now?

The weakness, wasting and fasciculation indicate involvement of lower motor neurons; the reflex changes and upgoing plantars mean that the disease is also affecting the upper motor neurons (in the corticospinal tracts). Therefore, his symptoms are not due a disease of muscle (such as polymyositis) or the neuromuscular junction (such as myasthenia gravis or Lambert–Eaton myasthenic syndrome).

Because of the upper motor neuron features, both multifocal motor neuropathy with conduction block and Kennedy's disease are unlikely; the absence of gynaecomastia also makes Kennedy's disease less likely. However, patients of this age often have a degree of cervical spondylitic disease, and the mixed picture could be explained by multifocal motor neuronopathy with conduction block occurring in the context of a cervical spondylitic myelopathy.

A mixed upper and lower motor neuron picture can be seen with a cervical spondylitic radiculomyelopathy, where age- or trauma-related degeneration of the cervical spine leads to compression of the exiting nerve roots (radiculopathy) and of the cord itself (myelopathy). However, the absence of any sensory features is against this, and the dysathria, the wasted and fasciculating tongue and the brisk jaw jerk imply that the nervous system is affected above the neck. Taken together, the findings are most in keeping with motor neuron disease (MND).

What investigations are required?

Routine blood tests are usually normal in MND, with the exception of a mild elevation of serum creatine kinase. Genetic testing is available to detect the expanded trinucleotide repeat in the androgen receptor gene that causes Kennedy's disease. Multifocal motor neuropathy with conduction block may be associated with IgM anti-

GM1 ganglioside antibodies. Imaging is usually normal, although MRI may show some atrophy of the corticospinal tracts in the pyramids. Importantly, MRI of the cervical spine often shows changes of cervical spondylitic disease in the age group commonly affected by MND, and it is important that such findings are not over-interpreted. The most important diagnostic test is the neurophysiological examination, where electromyography (EMG) shows changes of ongoing denervation (abnormal spontaneous activity such as fibrillation potentials), renervation, enlarged motor units and fasciculations. Nerve conduction studies show normal sensory nerve function and normal proximal motor conduction velocities (until late in the disease) but prolonged distal motor latencies. In contrast, in multifocal motor neuropathy, nerve conduction studies reveal multiple focal motor conduction blocks, slowed motor conduction, abnormal temporal dispersion and markedly prolonged F waves.

The patient returns to the clinic 4 weeks after first being seen. His creatine kinase was elevated at 216 units/L (normal range 38–174 units/L). MRI showed mild cervical spondylitic myelopathy only, and his EMG showed changes of active denervation with reinervation, enlarged motor units and electrical evidence of fasciculations in every muscle sampled. In the 4 weeks that elapsed since he had been seen there has been a marked progression both in his weakness and in his speech problems.

What causes motor neuron disease?

The aetiology of most cases of MND remains obscure. Between 2% and 5% of patients appear to have a familial form of MND, and of these about 20% are due to mutations in the SOD1 gene encoding superoxide dismutase, an enzyme involved in free radical scavenging. The genetic basis for the other 80% of familial cases, and the cause of the 95% of cases without a family history, is not known. However, it seems likely that the motor neuron lifespan is compromised by a combination of genetic and environmental factors.

How should patients with motor neuron disease be managed?
Organisation of care

As the disease progresses patients become more dependent on others in their activities of daily living, and develop increasing problems with mobility, swallowing and breathing. Often this progression can be rapid and unpredictable. Services for patients with motor neuron disease should therefore seek to coordinate the input of the many health professionals and social services involved; should seek to anticipate problems (for instance with respiratory function) before they become crises; and should inform and work with patients and their families to allow them to make informed choices about their management at every stage in their illness.

These functions are best served firstly by a Specialist Nurse Practitioner acting as a point of contact, providing information to the patient and their family, and coordinating the input of various other professionals; and secondly by the delivery of care in the context of a multidisciplinary outpatient clinic. In such a clinic there can be measurement of height, weight and respiratory parameters at presentation, the better to detect any later deterioration; opportunistic provision of, for example, dietary advice; and the opportunity for patients to discuss their future intentions and choices regarding respiratory support, enteral feeding and terminal care. While the organisation of care in this way does not prolong life, it does seem to increase quality of life.

Providing symptomatic relief

A major role of physiotherapy and occupational therapy is to maintain functional independence and independent mobility for as long as possible, partly through maximising what the patient can do and partly through adaptations to the environment. Important symptoms that are amenable to treatment include constipation (managed by a healthy diet, bulking agents and aperients), hypersalivation and drooling (which may be managed by hyoscine patches), and nocturnal aches and pains (which may be managed by amitryptiline).

Interventions to minimise complications

1 *Enteral feeding*: where nutritional status is impaired through dysphagia, this can be improved through the use of fortified drinks and yogurts. If this is not sufficient, or if the work of eating has become burdensome, or there is a risk of aspiration pneumonia, some patients do very well with percutaneous enteral feeding. This requires a degree of manual dexterity to attach and to use, so it is not suitable for patients who live alone and whose disease also affects their hand function.

2 *Respiratory support*: respiratory failure is a common mode of death in patients with MND, often in association with pneumonia. However, some patients have a degree of respiratory impairment through the night sufficient to cause daytime sleepiness and headache without an imminent risk of life-threatening respiratory failure. In these patients, nocturnal ventilation can lead to substantial improvement in the quality of that life that they have remaining.

Drug treatment

Riluzole blocks the tetradotoxin-sensitive sodium channel, thereby leading to reduced glutamate release and thence to reduced excitotoxicity. At a dose of 50 mg twice daily it probably prolongs life by a couple of months. Associated side effects include nausea and disrupted liver function tests.

Mr Patterson was seen by the MND multidisciplinary team, led by the MND Specialist Nurse. A dietary assessment showed a degree of malnutrition but normal swallowing, and he received dietary supplements. Respiratory function testing was within normal limits. A number of environmental home adaptations to prolong his functional independence were arranged. At review 3 months later he had continued to lose weight, he was choking on liquids and had daytime sleepiness and headaches. Further respiratory function testing showed a reduced vital capacity, with increased end-tidal CO_2 and overnight monitoring showed periods of hypoventilation with apnoeic episodes. After appropriate discussion he had a percutaneous endoscopic gastrostomy (PEG) tube placed and overnight ventilation. With this support he continued to enjoy a reasonable quality of life for a further 6 months, with occasional admissions to the hospice, before dying peacefully at home.

PART 2: CASES

CASE REVIEW

This 63-year-old man presented with a rapidly progressive weakness of the hands, then the legs and the bulbar muscles. On examination there were both upper and lower motor neuron features, and EMG confirmed the diagnosis of motor neuron disease. Despite a rapid clinical course, involvement of a multidisciplinary team substantially improved the quality of life in his remaining months.

KEY POINTS

- Even with untreatable, rapidly progressive neurological diseases, substantial improvements in the quality of remaining life can be achieved
- This is much better organised in the context of a multidisciplinary team
- The three pillars of intervention are environmental adaptation, dietary support and respiratory support
- Riluzole may prolong survival in patients with MND

Further reading and references

McDermott C, Shaw P. Clinical review. Diagnosis and management of motor neurone disease. *BMJ* 2008;**336**:658–62.

Case 22   A 55-year-old woman with episodes of excruciating facial pain

Mrs Mary Blackwood is a 55-year-old solicitor who reports 'excruciating pain' over the left side of her face. The episodes of pain last for a few seconds, arise from the corner of her mouth and shoot down her chin like 'electric shocks'. The pain is so severe that the discomfort often makes her jump. She avoids touching her face because this seems to make the sensations worse.

What causes of facial pain may be affecting Mrs Blackwood?

There are a number of potential causes of facial pain (Box 22.1). These include headache disorders, neuropathic pain syndromes, sinus and dental pathology, tempero-mandibular joint dysfunction and temporal arteritis.

Mrs Blackwood presented to her dentist as she wondered if her symptoms might be related to an underlying tooth abscess. Dental X-rays revealed a cracked tooth and she was prescribed a course of antibiotics. The episodes of pain persisted, however, and she went on to have the tooth extracted. Despite her tooth extraction, painful symptoms persisted and she was referred to a neurologist. A detailed clinical examination was unremarkable.

What is the most likely cause of this woman's painful facial sensory symptoms?

Momentary 'lancinating' pain occurring in the sensory distribution of the trigeminal nerve is highly suggestive of neuropathic pain. Trigeminal neuralgia is a neuropathic disorder arising due to irritation of the trigeminal nerve. The disorder affects approximately 1 in 10 000 people each year and tends to occur in people over the age of 55. Women are affected twice as often as men. As in this case, patients often describe an 'electric shock'-like, 'stabbing' or 'piercing' sensation. Painful symptoms last from seconds to minutes and arise particularly in the maxillary (V2) and mandibular (V3) divisions of the trigeminal nerve close to the nose or mouth.

What other features of the history are typical for this disorder?

Pain typically occurs paroxysmally in trigeminal neuralgia, frequently up to several times a day. Episodes may be sudden and severe, often causing the patient to jump, leading to the French term for the disorder, 'tic douloureux'. There may be a background dull ache and lancinating pain may be induced by contact with the skin of the affected area over so-called 'trigger zones'. Washing, shaving, brushing teeth, chewing, drinking, speaking and cold wind on the face may trigger symptoms and patients, therefore, avoid many of these activities. In severe cases patients may lose weight because of the pain experienced whilst chewing. The diagnostic criteria for trigeminal neuralgia are listed in Box 22.2.

Are there any investigations that may be of use at this stage?

The pain syndrome of trigeminal neuralgia is usually diagnosed from the history alone, and clinical examination is usually unremarkable in the 90–95% of patients with so-called 'idiopathic' disease. In some patients, pain may be associated with a brief facial spasm or tic. Pain is thought to arise as a result of irritation and compression of the proximal part of the trigeminal nerve by vascular structures in the posterior fossa such as a dilated, ectatic basilar artery or superior cerebellar artery, or arteriovenous anomalies. Other potential structural causes leading to compression of the trigeminal nerve roots along the pons include an arachnoid cyst, neuroma, meningioma or abnormalities of the skull base.

Trigeminal neuralgia is rare under the age of 40 years, and in patients with a younger age of onset, symptoms may represent a presentation of multiple sclerosis. If any

Neurology: Clinical Cases Uncovered, 1st edition. © M. Macleod, M. Simpson and S. Pal. Published 2011 by Blackwell Publishing Ltd.

Box 22.1 Common causes of facial pain

- Trigeminal neuralgia
- Glossopharyngeal neuralgia
- Post-herpetic neuralgia
- Dental pathology
- Temporal arteritis
- Sinus headache
- Temperomandibular joint dysfunction
- Facial migraine
- Cluster headache
- Primary stabbing ('ice pick') headache
- Trigeminal autonomic headache syndromes
- Chronic paroxysmal hemicranias

Box 22.2 Diagnostic criteria for trigeminal neuralgia

- Paroxysmal attacks of pain lasting from a fraction of a second to 2 minutes that affect one or more divisions of the trigeminal nerve
- Pain has at least one of the following characteristics:
  - intense, sharp, superficial or stabbing
  - pain may be precipitated by trigger areas, or trigger factors
  - attacks are similar in individual patients
- No neurological deficit is clinically evident
- Not attributed to another disorder

---

abnormal neurological signs are present, including loss of sensation over the face, MRI of the brain is indicated to exclude structural lesions and multiple sclerosis. Magnetic resonance angiography (MRA) may be of use in demonstrating blood vessels compressing the trigeminal nerve.

Mrs Blackwood's MRI brain scan showed no evidence of any vascular anomalies, structural pathology or demyelination. Despite reassurance that trigeminal neuralgia has no long-term sinister consequences she is extremely keen for any treatment that may help relieve the pain. She reports that symptoms have been getting her down lately and she has become low in mood.

What strategies may be employed in the management of her symptoms?

Patients with trigeminal neuralgia are often dismissed as having an underlying psychological aetiology to their symptoms and, as with many chronic pain syndromes, depression often coexists. Effective management includes patient education and reassurance that although symptoms may lead to avoidance of many activities of daily living, effective symptomatic treatments are available and, in most individuals, symptoms are not associated with sinister underlying neurological pathology. Trigeminal neuralgia tends to wax and wane spontaneously with symptoms occurring in cycles.

Eighty per cent of patients experience symptomatic benefit with medications alone. Complete spontaneous remissions may last for months to years and occur in 25% of cases. The relapse rate is approximately 1% per year. Opiate-based analgesia, however, generally offers little relief. Pain may be controlled pharmacologically with anticonvulsants like carbamazepine, lamotrigine or gabapentin. Phenytoin and sodium valproate can also be used. Baclofen is used as a second-line treatment.

Mrs Blackwood was provided with patient education leaflets and prescribed a course of carbamazepine. Her painful sensory symptoms settled and over time her mood improved accordingly.

What other interventions are employed for treatment when medications fail?

Other interventions for trigeminal neuralgia include radiofrequency ablation or phenol injection of the trigeminal ganglion, although both of these may lead to trigeminal sensory loss. Definitive treatment is by surgical decompression of the trigeminal nerve from a compressing vessel; however, this procedure carries the risks of posterior fossa surgery.

CASE REVIEW

Trigeminal neuralgia is a common cause of excruciating facial pain. Physical examination is usually unremarkable and patients are frequently misdiagnosed as having dental pathology or an underlying mood disorder. In the majority of cases no underlying structural cause is found and the disease is termed 'idiopathic'. In 5–10% of cases, underlying compression of the trigeminal nerve by a vascular anomaly, structural lesion or demyelination may be responsible for symptoms. The majority of patients respond very well to carbamazepine and surgical intervention may be reserved for refractory cases.

Further reading and references

Bennetto L, Patel NK, Fuller G. Trigeminal neuralgia and its management. *BMJ* 2007;**334**:201–5.

KEY POINTS

- Trigeminal neuralgia causes a characteristic lancinating facial pain syndrome
- The majority of cases are called 'idiopathic' but many are associated with vascular compression of the trigeminal nerve
- A minority of cases arise secondary to multiple sclerosis pathology or nerve compression by tumour
- Symptoms may cause patients to avoid activities of daily living that 'trigger' pain such as washing the face, shaving and even eating and drinking
- Most patients' symptoms respond well to drug treatments and carbamazepine is usually very effective
- If pharmacological intervention fails, successful surgical procedures are available including microvascular decompression

Case 23 A 38-year-old man with heaviness of the legs

Donald Adamson is a 38-year-old construction site manager. Over the past 8 weeks he has noticed 'heaviness' in his legs, particularly whilst climbing up stairs. During a recent holiday away with his family he noticed that he was struggling to lift his 3-year-old son up off the ground. Over the past 2 weeks he has struggled walking even short distances due to a feeling of 'tightness' in his thighs and calves. He has also noticed difficulties with a discomfort in his shoulders and arms when washing his hair, particularly the back of his head. Mr Adamson has been previously fit and well and takes no regular medications. He reports drinking approximately two bottles of wine per week. He has been otherwise systemically well with no weight loss, change in appetite or night sweats.

What thoughts run through your mind from Mr Adamson's history?

The history points to progressive difficulties in mobility and activities of daily living secondary to deteriorating weakness which has occurred over weeks (subacute). The weakness appears to be symmetrical and affecting both arms and legs. There is no mention of double vision, speech or swallowing problems. No sensory symptoms are reported, nor are there symptoms of sphincter dysfunction. Whilst it is possible his symptoms may be due to an upper motor neuron lesion, such a lesion would need to be affecting both cerebral hemispheres or somewhere high up in the cervical cord. A lower motor neuron pathology, affecting the nerve, muscle or neuromuscular junction is, therefore, more likely.

On examination the muscles around his shoulder, thighs and calves are tender on palpation. He has normal muscle bulk and tone in the limbs. On testing power, neck flexion, shoulder abduction and hip flexion can all be overcome in a

symmetrical manner. His reflexes are all present. On further testing it is apparent Mr Adamson has difficulty rising from a low chair and is unable to do so without using his arms for support.

What sort of neurological process does Mr Adamson's examination suggest?

The examination findings indicate a lower motor neuron pattern of weakness. Proximal symmetrical weakness with no sensory deficits and no mention of bladder or bowel symptoms makes a disorder of muscles (myopathy) most likely.

What other questions are relevant to ask Mr Adamson?

1 Are muscles aching and tender? If so, this is suggestive of muscle inflammation or necrosis.

2 Is there any change in the colour of urine being passed? Darkened urine (tea or cola coloured) suggests myoglobinuria.

3 Do symptoms of weakness fluctuate or worsen as the day progresses? If so, this is suggestive of a myasthenia gravis, a disorder affecting the neuromuscular junction.

4 Are there any sensory or bladder and bowel symptoms? If these are present, this makes disease of the muscle much less likely.

5 Have there been any symptoms of palpitations or breathlessness suggestive of pulmonary oedema? Many disorders of skeletal muscle also result in cardiomyopathies.

Mr Adamson's muscles are tender and the discomfort is worse on squeezing them. His symptoms are worse after exertion but do not fluctuate as the day progresses. He reports no sensory symptoms and no symptoms of bladder or bowel dysfunction. His urine has not changed in colour and there are no cardiac symptoms of note.

Neurology: Clinical Cases Uncovered, 1st edition. © M. Macleod, M. Simpson and S. Pal. Published 2011 by Blackwell Publishing Ltd.

Box 23.1 Common causes of myopathies

Inflammatory myopathies
- Polymyositis:
  - most common inflammatory muscle disease in adults: 6 per 100 000
  - especially common in women, 30–60 years
  - onset is usually subacute/chronic
  - proximal limb, trunk, neck, pharyngeal and oesophageal muscles: painful or tender
- Dermatomyositis:
  - often more severe and acute
  - myositis + purple 'heliotrope' rash around the eyes + linear rash over knuckles and proximal phalanges: Gottron's papules
- Inclusion body myositis:
  - commonest inflammatory muscle disorder in middle-aged men
  - slowly progressive, affecting specific muscles in early stages, e.g. brachioradialis
- Sarcoidosis

Metabolic and endocrine myopathies
- Thyroid disease (hyper-/hypothyroid)
- Cushing's syndrome
- Addison's disease
- Acromegaly
- Hypo-/hyperkalaemia
- Hypomagnesaemia
- Hypocalcaemia
- Diabetes mellitus
- Liver
- Renal failure

Drug- and toxin-induced myopathies
- Steroids
- Cocaine
- Heroin
- Antiretrovirals
- Ciclosporin
- Opiates
- Statins
- Beta-blockers
- Penicillamine
- Organophosphates
- Alcohol
- Halothane general anaesthetics (leading to malignant hyperthermia)

Hereditary myopathies
- Muscular dystrophies (MDs):
  - Duchenne's MD
  - Becker's MD
  - facioscapulohumeral MD
  - limb girdle MD
  - Emery–Dreifuss MD
  - oculopharyngeal MD
- Myotonic syndromes:
  - myotonic dystrophy
- Metabolic myopathies:
  - mitochondrial myopathy
  - McArdle's disease
- Non-progressive congenital myopathies
- Syndromes of episodic weakness or periodic paralysis
- Myotonia congenita, paramyotonia congenital, periodic paralysis

Infectious myopathies
- Trichinosis
- Toxoplasmosis
- HIV
- Coxsackie viruses
- Influenza
- Lyme disease

What are the common causes of myopathic disease?

Causes of myopathy can be categorised into six main groups (Box 23.1): (1) inflammatory, (2) endocrine and metabolic, (3) drug and toxin induced, (4) hereditary, and (5) infectious.

What investigations are appropriate at this stage?

Initial blood tests for investigating Mr Anderson's suspected myopathy include a full blood count (FBC), urea and electrolytes (U&E), thyroid function tests (TFTs), erythrocyte sedimentation rate (ESR) and a creatinine kinase (CK) level. Other blood tests to consider include serum cortisol, lactate, antinuclear antibody (ANA), antinuclear cytoplasmic antibody (ANCA) and angiotensin-converting enzyme (ACE).

Mr Anderson's blood tests were all grossly normal apart from a CK of 13 800 IU/L.

What other tests are worth considering at this point?

The following investigations were also performed:

- *Normal ECG*
- *Normal echocardiogram*
- *Electromyography (EMG) demonstrating abnormal, short duration, polyphasic motor unit potentials*
- *Muscle biopsy demonstrating evidence of necrosis of muscle fibres with vacuoles*

What diagnosis does the history, examination and investigation results suggest?

The history and examination findings are suggestive of a myopathic process. The grossly elevated CK (normal levels <200 IU/L) suggest an inflammatory process with muscle necrosis. This is confirmed by the EMG and muscle biopsy results. The normal ECG and echocardiogram demonstrate there is no evidence of an associated cardiomyopathy or cardiac conduction defect.

Inflammatory myopathies such as polymyositis and dermatomyositis frequently have an autoimmune basis and present with systemic symptoms prior to the onset of proximal weakness. There is no evidence of this with Mr Anderson. Furthermore, whilst these disorders may occur in isolation, they frequently arise as part of a widespread collagen–vascular disease. Mr Anderson has no skin rash and no evidence of bulbar involvement affecting speech, swallowing or breathing. Furthermore, there is an increased risk of neoplasia, especially lymphoma and ovarian cancer with polymyositis (6% of cases) and dermatomyositis (15% of cases) and there is no evidence for this in Mr Anderson's case.

Routine blood tests have excluded a metabolic or endocrine cause of the myopathy and the older age of onset of symptoms and lack of family history point away from an inherited myopathy. He is not taking any regular medications or recreational drugs that may contribute to a toxic myopathy.

Further questioning revealed Mr Anderson had recently felt under immense pressure at work and had started binging on whisky at weekends. Quantification of his intake suggested he had recently been drinking up to 70 units of alcohol a week.

The exclusion of other causes of a myopathy in conjunction with this additional history led to a diagnosis of acute alcoholic myopathy. In addition to the acute syndrome of muscle necrosis, alcohol causes a more chronic myopathy associated with gradual progressive weakness and atrophy that usually involves the hip and shoulder girdle. This chronic myopathy does not result in myoglobinuria or elevated creatine kinase levels.

What potential renal complication results from an acute inflammatory myopathy?

Acute muscle necrosis may result in precipitation of myoglobin in the renal tubules and can cause acute renal tubular necrosis.

How is this avoided?

Aggressive hydration with intravenous fluids and, occasionally, diuretics are essential to maintain renal function.

What are the potential complications of a myopathic disease in general?

Patients with myopathic disease are predisposed to swallowing difficulties and respiratory failure. Many specific myopathies are associated with cardiac arrhythmias, hypertension, gastric dilation, endocrinopathies and cataracts.

What treatments are commonly used for myopathies?

Treatment of inflammatory myopathies is often with corticosteroids and other forms of immunosuppression such as intravenous immunoglobulin and azathioprine. In cases of toxic myopathies, withdrawal of the offending agent, for example drugs or alcohol, may lead to spontaneous reversal of inflammatory changes.

Mr Anderson was treated with intravenous fluids. Urinalysis revealed the presence of myoglobunuria but his renal function remained stable. He was counselled regarding the acute and chronic complications of drinking excess alcohol and referred to local support services. His symptoms gradually improved over the next 10 days and his CK levels also returned to normal in this period of time.

CASE REVIEW

This middle-aged man presented with a short history of progressive weakness of the proximal muscles in the legs, arms and trunk. There were no sensory symptoms or signs and no features suggestive of myasthenia. CK, EMG and muscle biopsy were all consistent with a toxic necrotising myopathy, but there was no inflammatory infiltrate on biopsy such as might be seen in an inflammatory myositis. Re-taking the history suggested that a recent dramatic increase in alcohol intake might be responsible, and when he stopped drinking his symptoms abated rapidly.

Further reading and references

Merrison AF, Hanna MG. Neurology in practice. The bare essentials: muscle disease. *Pract Neurol* 2009;**9**:54–65.

KEY POINTS

- Myopathies typically lead to proximal, symmetrical weakness without sensory deficits or sphincter disturbance
- Patients often describe difficulty rising from a sitting or squatting position and difficulties lifting their arms above their head
- Myopathies can be classified as inflammatory, endocrine and metabolic, drug and toxin induced, hereditary or infectious
- Important investigations include CK level, inflammatory markers, endocrine and metabolic screens as well as EMG and a muscle biopsy
- Many inflammatory myopathies can be treated successfully with steroids or other immunomodulatory drugs

Case 24 An 84-year-old man with confusion and unsteadiness

Bert, an 84-year-old man, is brought to the emergency department by the police after having been picked up wandering naked down the main street. When questioned, he stated that he was looking for his mother.

What are the key features of the history and examination?

This patient presents with a confusional state, one of the commonest reasons for presentation to the emergency department. The list of possible causes is vast, and a careful and methodical approach is therefore required.

1 What is the duration of his confusional state?
   • Acute vs subacute vs chronic. Collateral history from family, friends, GP or anyone who knows the patient is essential in this case as the patient's ability to give a history is limited.
2 What is his past medical (including psychiatric) history and drug history? Again, collateral history is mandatory.
3 Is there a history of head injury?
4 Are there any systemic symptoms?
5 Is the patient febrile or are there signs of systemic infection or hypoxia?
6 Is he hypoglycaemic?
7 Are there any focal neurological findings?

The emergency department nurses find a card in his wallet with his address and call his home, but there is no reply. The House Officer calls his GP who says that he has not seen Bert for 2 years and the last time he presented was with an ingrown toenail. He has not been supplying him with any medication and as far as he knows the patient has

not been in hospital before. He does not have any relatives and the only place he goes regularly is the corner shop to buy his food. The House Officer, who is very efficient, calls the corner shop owner and she states that he used to be very sharp, and would always remember the things on his shopping list, but over the past month he has been confused and has sometimes come in twice or three times in the day to buy the same set of shopping.

This history suggests a subacute confusional state, with a duration of several weeks. There are no clues from the history as to its aetiology and a careful examination is necessary

On examination, he is alert and cooperative but confused and disorientated to time and place, and appears unkempt, but there is no evidence of dysphasia or dysarthria. He is afebrile and oxygen saturations are 99% on room air. His heart rate is 80 beats/min and regular, and his blood pressure is 140/90 mmHg. Examination of the cardiovascular, respiratory and abdominal systems is unremarkable. On neurological examination, the visual fields are full, eye movements are normal and there is no facial weakness. Examination of tone, power, coordination and reflexes in the limbs is also normal on the bed, but when the patient tries to walk he is unsteady and falls over.

What is the likely differential diagnosis now?

The patient is confused and unsteady without other focal findings on neurological examination, and there is no clinical evidence of systemic illness to account for his confusion. The differential diagnosis is therefore very wide (Box 24.1).

What is the appropriate plan of investigation and management?

Because of the wide variety of possible causes, the patient requires the following baseline investigations:

Neurology: Clinical Cases Uncovered, 1st edition. © M. Macleod, M. Simpson and S. Pal. Published 2011 by Blackwell Publishing Ltd.

Box 24.1 Differential diagnosis of an acute or subacute confusional state in the elderly

Structural brain lesions
- Stroke
- Brain tumour (benign, malignant primary or metastases)
- Subdural haematoma (acute or chronic)
- Subarachnoid haemorrhage
- Normal pressure hydrocephalus
- Cerebral vasculitis

Neurodegenerative processes
- Alzheimer's disease
- Lewy body dementia
- Frontotemporal dementia
- Creutzfeldt–Jakob disease

Systemic causes
- Infection (most commonly urinary tract or respiratory, but also need to consider CNS infection – meningitis/ encephalitis)
- Medication side effect or poisoning
- Drug or alcohol withdrawal
- Renal failure/uraemia
- Hepatic encephalopathy
- Hypoxaemia
- Electrolyte disturbance (particularly hyponatraemia, hypocalcaemia)
- Metabolic disturbance (hypothyroidism)
- B12 deficiency
- Thiamine deficiency (Wernicke–Korsakoff syndrome)
- Syphilis
- HIV
- Carbon monoxide poisoning

Psychiatric causes
- Depression
- Psychosis

1 Blood tests:
- Glucose (most urgent, because hypoglycaemic brain damage can be permanent and is rapidly correctable)
- Full blood count (looking for evidence of infection or anaemia)
- Urea and electrolytes (looking for evidence of renal failure or hypo-/hypernatraemia in particular)
- Liver function tests (looking for evidence of systemic malignancy or hepatic failure)
- Thyroid function tests
- B12 and folate levels

2 Chest X-ray: respiratory tract infection and lung malignancy are common causes of confusion and must be excluded in confused patients, particularly if there are signs of fever, hypoxia or a history of smoking or any respiratory symptoms.

3 Brain imaging: especially if no clear cause is found from the routine blood tests. The patient requires imaging with a plain CT scan to exclude a neoplasm, stroke or subdural haematoma.

4 Medication review: it is essential to review the patient's medication history, in particular looking for new medications or medications that have been changed recently.

5 Other investigations: the following investigations should also be considered:
- Lumbar puncture (looking for evidence of encephalitis, meningitis, subarachnoid haemorrhage or malignant infiltration of the CSF)
- MRI scan of the brain (looking in more detail for structural lesions, stroke or changes of encephalitis or atrophy which may indicate a chronic neurodegenerative process)
- Blood testing for coagulation profile, HIV, syphilis, paracetamol/salicylate levels, autoimmune diseases or thiamine deficiency (red cell transketolase) – although if the latter is even suspected, empirical treatment with thiamine and B vitamins is mandatory, without waiting for confirmatory test results

Routine blood tests were performed that showed a normal glucose, full blood count and normal liver function tests. Renal function was normal but serum sodium was reduced to 129 mmol/L. The House Officer ordered a CT scan of the brain (Fig. 24.1).

What is the diagnosis?

The CT scan (Fig. 24.1) shows bilateral, crescent-shaped extra-axial hypodense collections of chronic subdural haematoma. This occurs as a result of venous bleeding from the bridging veins from the cortex to the superior sagittal sinus. In the acute stages of bleeding, i.e. the first 3 days, the haematoma appears hyperdense (bright-coloured) on CT, and subsequently becomes isodense and then hypodense (darker) after around 3 weeks.

Acute subdural haemorrhage occurs as a result of traumatic brain injury, either due to blunt trauma (in which case the bleed is often on the contrecoup side, opposite to the site of injury) or in association with deceleration or rotational injury, without an actual impact (see Case 14).

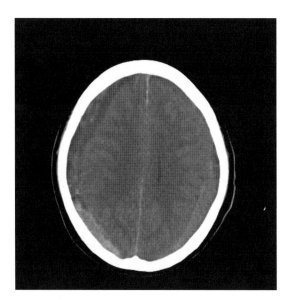

Figure 24.1 CT of the brain showing chronic subdural haematoma in this patient.

The cause of chronic subdural haemorrhage is often more difficult to identify, and often there is no definite history of trauma. They are more common in the older population (where the bridging veins are more fragile) and in alcoholics; other predisposing factors include coagulopathies (including warfarin therapy), seizures, CSF shunts and any condition that puts the patient at risk of falls.

Presentation of subdural haemorrhage is variable. Presenting symptoms can include hemiparesis, hemineglect, dysphasia, altered mental status or decreased conscious level. Acute subdural haemorrhage may cause a significant midline shift and may require urgent surgical decompression to prevent transtorial herniation (or 'coning') and death. Chronic subdural haemorrhage, by contrast, may be well tolerated or even asymptomatic.

What is the management of subdural haemorrhage?

Acute subdural haemorrhage may require urgent surgical treatment with decompression through an open craniotomy or through burr hole drainage. Chronic subdural haemorrhage, if asymptomatic, may not necessarily require treatment, and a 'watch and wait' approach may be adopted instead. If symptomatic, surgical drainage through burr holes or craniotomy is required.

Bert remains confused and at times appears drowsy. The neurosurgeons evacuate the subdural through burr holes in the skull, and his confusion gradually improves. He is eventually able to leave hospital and moves to a sheltered housing where he takes up a position as a bingo caller.

CASE REVIEW

After careful chasing of the available history, it becomes clear that this patient has a subacute confusional state, the causes of which are legion. The treating doctors must adopt a methodical and careful approach to the examination and investigations, ruling out each of these possible causes. In this case, history, examination and blood tests did not reveal any definite cause (the reduced sodium is likely to be a consequence of the subdural haemorrhage rather than a cause of confusion itself) and it is the CT scan which provides the diagnosis. In this case, surgical treatment of the subdural haemorrhage was indicated because of persisting confusion and drowsiness.

KEY POINTS

- Confused patients are unable to give an accurate history themselves, therefore it is essential to obtain all possible information from other sources
- The list of possible causes of confusion is wide and the treating doctor must bear these in mind when examining the patient and formulating a plan of investigations
- Subdural haemorrhage may be acute or chronic; the duration and severity of symptoms determine when and whether surgical evacuation is required

Further reading and references

Adhiyaman V, Asghar M, Ganeshram KN, Bhowmick BK. Chronic subdural haematoma in the elderly. *Postgrad Med J* 2002;**78**(916):71–5.

Case 25 A 45-year-old man with constant headache

Joshua is a 45-year-old businessman who has been referred to neurology outpatients with a headache. It is present almost constantly, and he is at the end of his tether. His business partner recently died of a brain tumour and he is becoming increasingly worried that this will happen to him.

What are the key features of the history?

The headache history should begin with an open question (e.g. 'tell me about your headaches') followed by a period of time for the patient to describe their symptoms and raise their concerns. This should be followed up with specific questions designed to gather the following information:

1 What is the duration of the headache?
2 Is it episodic or constant? What is its periodicity?
3 What are its location, severity and character?
4 Are there any associated symptoms?
   • Focal limb weakness or sensory symptoms
   • Visual disturbance
   • Speech disturbance
   • Seizures
   • Personality change
   • Lacrimation
5 Are there any exacerbating factors?
   • Coughing
   • Sneezing
   • Bending over
   • Valsalva manoeuvre
   • Chewing
   • Cold weather
6 *Exactly* what medications (prescribed and over-the-counter) is he taking and when? Do they work, and if so for how long?
7 How much caffeine is he consuming?

Neurology: Clinical Cases Uncovered, 1st edition. © M. Macleod, M. Simpson and S. Pal. Published 2011 by Blackwell Publishing Ltd.

8 Does he have any systemic symptoms that might suggest underlying malignancy or other pathology?

Joshua has had the headache for almost 9 months. Initially it was present around three times per week, but has gradually become more frequent, and it is now almost constant. It is localised to the front of his head, and is usually about 3/10 severity, although it can be worse before he takes the painkillers. There are no associated symptoms, and he has not identified any exacerbating factors. The only thing that helps are the strong paracetamol/codeine tablets, which take the edge off his pain thus enabling him to work, but he is always watching the clock to see when his next painkillers are due, and he does not feel they are helping him as much as they used to. His headaches are noticeably worse before the first coffee of the day, and he is currently drinking up to 8 cups in an average day at work. He has been feeling anxious since his business partner died and he has not been sleeping well, but denies any other symptoms on systemic enquiry. Neurological examination, including fundoscopy, was normal, and a CT scan of brain was also normal.

What is the diagnosis?

Joshua describes a chronic, daily headache, with no features of migraine (see Case 20). Initially the headache was episodic but is now constant, and he is using analgesia on a daily basis. The neurologist first has to decide whether this is a primary headache disorder or a headache that is secondary to neurological or systemic disease. The duration of the headache, the absence of any precipitating or accompanying features, the normal clinical examination, the normal CT scan and the absence of any other findings on clinical examination argue strongly in favour of a primary headache disorder.

This patient has a combination of tension-type headache (headache without features of migraine or any of the other headache syndromes; Box 25.1) and medication overuse headache. He has headaches on more than

---

Box 25.1 International Headache Society classification

Primary headache disorders
- Migraine
  - migraine without aura
  - migraine with aura
- Tension-type headache
  - infrequent episodic tension-type headache
  - frequent episodic tension-type headache
  - chronic tension-type headache
- Trigeminal autonomic cephalalgias
  - Cluster headache
  - SUNCT syndrome (short-lived, unilateral headache with conjunctival injection and tearing)
  - paroxysmal hemicrania
- Other primary headache disorders
  - primary cough headache
  - primary sex headache
  - hypnic headache
  - hemicrania continua

Secondary headaches
- Trauma (head and/or neck)
- Subarachnoid haemorrhage
- Subdural haematoma
- Stroke
- Giant cell arteritis
- Meningitis/encephalitis
- Raised intracranial pressure
- Space-occupying lesion (brain tumour, abscess)
- Idiopathic intracranial hypertension
- Acute hydrocephalus
- Alcohol
- Carbon dioxide retention
- Carbon monoxide poisoning
- Medication overuse
- Hypertensive crisis
- Cervicogenic headache
- Acute glaucoma

---

15 days per month, therefore this is defined as *chronic* rather than *episodic* tension-type headache. His frequent use of painkillers constitutes medication overuse headache. The International Headache Society defines medication overuse as over 10 days per month for ergots, triptans and opiates, and over 15 days per month for simple analgesics and non-steroidal anti-inflammatory drugs (NSAIDs).

What causes tension-type headache?

Tension headache is often associated with emotional or psychosocial stress, although a causal link has not been proven, and the frequency of exogenous stressors is no different between chronic tension-type headache and chronic migraine. The pathophysiological mechanism behind the pain is poorly understood. Various mechanisms have been proposed, including nociceptor sensitisation by peripherally released inflammatory mediators, and abnormalities in central nociceptive processing, with decreased pain thresholds in patients with chronic tension-type headache.

What is the best management for tension-type headache?

Episodic tension-type headache can be effectively treated by simple analgesics, however care must be taken to avoid frequent analgesic use as this may precipitate medication overuse headache. Many non-drug therapies

have been used, including greater occipital nerve injection, acupuncture and other complimentary medicines. While acupuncture has been shown to improve symptoms, at least in the short term, no convincing randomized trial evidence for other non-drug therapies exists.

Amitriptyline, a tricyclic antidepressant, has been shown to be effective in the prophylaxis of chronic tension-type headache, as well as migraine, although the mechanism of action is not fully understood. The selective serotonin receptor inhibitors such as fluoxetine have not been shown to be effective in tension headache without associated depression. Powerful analgesics and opiates are not indicated and may worsen the situation by precipitating medication overuse headache. Prophylactic medications will *not* be effective if the patient is concurrently overusing analgesia on an 'as required' basis.

What is the management for medication overuse headache?

Medication overuse can be a problem with all analgesics including simple analgesics, ergot agents and opioids. Caffeine intake can also contribute to this problem. The only effective management is analgesic withdrawal, and this can be done safely as an outpatient in most cases, with the use of a medication diary, provided patients are sufficiently educated about the process. Patients must be well hydrated and may require a period of absence from work.

The original headache (which led to the medication overuse) will usually return, however it can be managed more effectively with prophylactic medications.

The neurologist diagnoses tension-type headache with superadded medication overuse headache. Joshua understands the importance of stopping his medication and, with support from his GP and the use of a medication diary, manages to cut out the co-codamol and to reduce his medication intake dramatically. He attends bereavement counselling in relation to the death of his business partner and is commenced on prophylactic treatment for tension-type headache with amitriptyline; at his 6-month review appointment his background headache is gone and he is having episodic headaches around once a month.

CASE REVIEW

The patient presents with a chronic daily headache without migrainous features and without other neurological symptoms. He is using strong painkillers on a daily basis. This suggests a diagnosis of chronic tension-type headache together with medication overuse headache. He was managed with medication withdrawal together with the introduction of prophylactic medication, and bereavement counselling in relation to the psychological stressors that exacerbated his original headache, and has a good outcome.

KEY POINTS

- The majority of headaches seen in neurology outpatients are primary headache disorders, although it is important not to miss headaches secondary to intracranial or systemic disease
- Many patients with chronic headache have additional problems with medication overuse, which exacerbates the problem
- Management of chronic headache is holistic, and involves withdrawal of medication as well as addressing psychological factors that may be contributing to the headache

Further reading and references

Loder E, Rizzoli P. Tension-type headache. *BMJ* 2008;**336** (7635):88–92.

Case 26 A 68-year-old man with a 2-week history of unsteadiness

Edward Roberts is a 68-year-old farmer who presents following a 2-week history of unsteadiness whilst walking, first noticed during a holiday in Amsterdam. His wife noticed that he seemed to be bumping into things. Mr Roberts commented that he did not see things as well on his right side. Over the past few days he has been having difficulties concentrating and feels that he is increasingly forgetful. He has also begun to experience a headache in the mornings which is worse when he coughs or sneezes. Mr Roberts' past medical history includes hypertension and he also had a melanoma removed from the left side of his abdomen 3 years ago.

What do you think is causing Mr Roberts' symptoms?

Neurological symptoms have come on and progressed rapidly over 2 weeks. A sudden onset of symptoms may suggest a vascular aetiology such as a stroke. A subacute deterioration suggests an inflammatory, infective or neoplastic process affecting the central nervous system. The history of new-onset unsteadiness, visual disturbance and morning headache are suspicious of a space-occupying lesion.

On examination there is no evidence of lymphadenopathy. His Mini-Mental State Examination score is 25/30 with deficits in orientation and concentration. Examination of his fundi reveals blurring of his optic disc suggestive of papilloedema on the left. Visual field testing reveals a right homonomous hemianopia. He has difficulties walking in a straight line and does appear to bump into objects on his right.

Where do you think the underlying lesion may be?

The examination findings add weight to the suspicion of an underlying space-occupying lesion. Difficulties with

balance may localise the lesion to the posterior fossa but a large space-occupying lesion in any region may results in gait unsteadiness. His reports of not being able to see things very well to his right suggests he may have a visual field defect. Memory problems suggest an underlying lesion in the temporal lobes. Mr Roberts may have one or several lesions to explain his symptoms.

If Mr Roberts does have a space-occupying lesion, what are the likely causes?

Intracranial space-occupying lesions can be caused by tumours, abscesses, haematomas, large aneurysms and arteriovenous malformations. The history and examination findings are most suggestive of an intracranial tumour. Intracranial neoplasms can be divided into primary tumours or more commonly occurring secondary intracranial metastases. Tumours can also be classified as intrinsic (within the substance of the brain) or extrinsic (occurring outside of the brain substance, most commonly the meninges). Intracranial tumours are more common in children than in adults and the pattern of tumours differs in that in adults 75% of tumours are supratentorial whereas in children 75% are infratentorial.

Which are the most common intrinsic and extrinsic brain tumours?

The most common tumours are outlined in Table 26.1.

What investigations would you perform next?

Neuroimaging is the key test for investigating the nature of Mr Roberts' underlying lesion. MRI of the brain will demonstrate over 95% of intracranial tumours. Most patients will have a CT scan of the head in the first instance due to greater access to this form of scanning. The differential diagnosis can be narrowed considerably by the site and appearance of the lesion.

Neurology: Clinical Cases Uncovered, 1st edition. © M. Macleod, M. Simpson and S. Pal. Published 2011 by Blackwell Publishing Ltd.

Table 26.1 Common intrinsic and extrinsic brain tumours.

Intrinsic tumours	Extrinsic tumours
Cerebral metastases	Meningioma
Gliobastoma multiforme	Pituitary adenoma
Astrocytoma	Schwannoma
Oligodendroglioma	
Ependymoma	

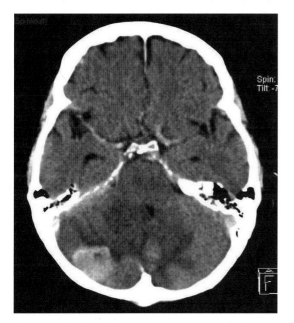

Figure 26.1 CT of the head showing an occipital mass with surrounding oedema in this patient.

Mr Roberts' scan demonstrates an abnormal lesion in the left occipital cortex with surrounding mass effect (Fig. 26.1).

What is the most likely diagnosis?

The neuroimaging appearances are of an intrinsic tumour, most probably a solitary metastasis. Given Mr Roberts' past medical history, metastatic melanoma is the most likely diagnosis.

Which other tumours commonly metastasise to brain?

Other primary tumours that metastasise to brain include cancers of the lung, breast and bowel.

How should management proceed next?

A clear and frank discussion with Mr Roberts is required at this point. In particular, he needs to be made aware that his neurological symptoms are secondary to a tumour in the brain and that this is likely to have arisen as a result of recurrence and spread of melanoma. A multidisiplinary team approach is crucial, with involvement of a clinical nurse specialist in oncology, neuro-oncologists, neuroradiologists, neurosurgeons and radiation and chemotherapy oncologists.

Cerebral oedema related to the tumour may respond temporarily to steroid therapy, usually dexamethasone. Treatment with steroids often results in dramatic improvement of headache and may even result in transient improvement of balance in Mr Roberts' case.

In patients where a primary cancer is not known, tissue biopsy is mandatory for establishing a diagnosis.

What other complications may emerge?

Tumours involving the cerebral cortex or hippocampus may result in epilepsy. Anticonvulsants are, therefore, often used prophylactically. As patients become immobile they become at risk of venous thrombosis.

What is the role of chemotherapy, radiotherapy and surgery?

Systemic cancers that have metastasised to the brain are generally incurable and treatment is directed at preventing disability and suffering. Radiation is the primary treatment of brain metastases. Where multiple metastases are present, whole brain irradiation is often employed. Focal or stereotactic radiotherapy can be administered to isolated lesions. When a single metastasis is present, as in Mr Roberts' case, surgical excision can be performed as a palliative measure. If the systemic cancer is treated appropriately and under control, resection of a single metastasis can improve survival and minimise disability. Survival appears improved when surgery is followed by whole brain radiotherapy. As a general rule, metastases do not respond to chemotherapy as well as primary brain tumours. Some cases, however, do experience dramatic improvement with systemic chemotherapy or hormonal therapies.

CT of the chest, abdomen and pelvis showed evidence of liver and lung metastases thought typical of melanoma, and this was confirmed following biopsy of one of the liver lesions. He began a course of chemotherapy, but continued to decline rapidly and died 7 weeks after diagnosis.

CASE REVIEW

This elderly man presented with a past history of melanoma and a short history of ataxia and mild cognitive impairment. CT scanning showed a lesion in the left occipital lobe with surrounding cerebral oedema and with significant mass effect, consistent with either a primary CNS tumour such as a glioma or with metastatic disease. Systemic investigation and biopsy confirmed the diagnosis of metastatic melanoma.

KEY POINTS

- Patients with rapidly progressive, focal neurological impairment need urgent assessment and imaging, if only to let them know what their future might hold
- Tumours commonly metastasising to the CNS include melanoma and tumours of the breast, kidney, lung and bowel
- While steroids may temporarily reverse some of the symptoms and signs associated with CNS tumours, this is usually a temporary phenomenon
- Tumour-associated epilepsy is a major source of morbidity in patients dying with CNS tumours

Further reading and references

Wen PY, Kesari S. Medical progress: malignant gliomas in adults. *N Engl J Med* 2008;**359**:492–507.

A 15-year-old girl with fidgeting movements

Kirsty Allen is a 15-year-old student who presents with fidgeting movements of the left side of her face, arm and leg. The movements seem to flow continuously in fits from the face to the leg but in a random pattern. She has no control over the movements but they do appear to get worse when she is anxious. She is rather embarrassed by the movements and they have affected her ability to take part in sports at school. Kirsty is otherwise fit and well with no significant past medical problems other than asthma for which she takes a salbutamol inhaler. She remembers having a severe throat infection a couple of months ago.

Which parts of the nervous system are typically responsible for involuntary movements?

Abnormal involuntary movements are referred to in neurology as 'movement disorders'. These movements do not usually arise as a result of weakness or sensory deficits but usually as a result of pathology affecting the basal ganglia or cerebellum, otherwise referred to as the extrapyramidal motor system.

How would you assess and classify Kirsty's movement disorder?

A simple way of thinking of movement disorders is to divide them into 'hyperkinesias', which involve an excess of movement, or 'hypokinesias', which involve a reduction of movement. Kirsty's movements sound like hyperkinesia. It is important to take time to stand back and observe Kirsty's abnormal movements and describe what you see. Some patients may be self-conscious and try and inhibit their movements, particularly if these are embarrassing. Patients must, therefore, be put at ease as much as possible.

Neurology: Clinical Cases Uncovered, 1st edition. © M. Macleod, M. Simpson and S. Pal. Published 2011 by Blackwell Publishing Ltd.

Kirsty has abnormal involuntary fidgeting, writhing and twitching movements affecting the left side of her face, arm and leg. The movements appear semi-purposeful.

How else can abnormal movements be described?

Several types of abnormal movement disorder have been described, including the following:

1 *Akathisia*: a subjective feeling of inner restlessness which is relieved by movement. This movement disorder may result following treatment with psychiatric medications, particularly neuroleptics.
2 *Athetosis*: slow, sinuous, writhing movements usually involving the distal parts of the limbs.
3 *Ballismus*: wild, flinging, flailing, large amplitude movements of a limb. This may arise in one limb in which case it is termed hemiballismus.
4 *Chorea*: semi-purposeful flowing movements that flit from one body part to another in a continuous random pattern.
5 *Dyskinesia*: a general term used for any excessive movement. Dyskinesias are often seen as a complication of treatment in Parkinson's disease with levodopa.
6 *Myoclonus*: sudden, brief, shock-like jerks.
7 *Tremor*: rhythmic oscillatory movements that may be present at rest or with action.

All of the common abnormal movements may be caused by drugs, including neuroleptics, levodopa, lithium and anticonvulsants.

Kirsty's abnormal movements are choreiform.

What general medical conditions may cause chorea?

Chorea may arise in hyperthyroidism, during pregnancy, with the oral contraceptive pill, following the use of neuroleptic drugs and with systemic lupus erythematosus (SLE).

Kirsty's routine blood tests, thyroid function tests and blood tests for SLE were all normal. There was no history of neuroleptic drug use. Her oral contraceptive pill was stopped but her abnormal movements persisted.

Do you know of any inherited forms of chorea?

Huntington's disease (HD) is an autosomal, dominantly inherited disorder that leads to a progressive movement disorder associated with dementia and psychiatric symptoms. Most patients develop symptoms between the ages of 30 and 60 and can develop chorea affecting the tongue, face, trunk and limbs. Dystonia (twisting movements or movements that are sustained for variable periods of time) may also be present, as may tics (repetitive stereotyped movements or sounds that are suppressible and that seem to relieve a feeling of inner tension). A change in personality, disinhibition, depression and psychosis may also be apparent.

What diagnostic tests are there for Huntington's disease?

A detailed family history is important for diagnosing HD. A CT or MRI scan of the brain may demonstrate atrophy of the caudate nuclei. The diagnosis can be made genetically by finding an expanded trinucleotide CAG repeat on the short arm of chromosome 4. Patients with a family history of the disease can now be tested presymptomatically to discover whether they carry the gene. Because of the serious implications of positive genetic testing, both for the individual (whether yet affected by HD or not) and for other family members, a full and frank discussion is required prior to testing. Where the test has diagnostic implications for other family members (for instance where a grandparent was affected and the relevant parent is asymptomatic and does not wish to know their HD status), involvement of genetic counselling services can be exceptionally helpful.

What treatments are there for Huntington's disease?

HD is progressive and treatment is currently aimed at controlling symptoms. Tetrabenazine and haloperidol may help with abnormal movements.

A detailed family history reveals that no-one in Kirsty's family experienced similar movements or died early from a neurological or psychiatric illness. Examination reveals no cognitive deficits and she has no psychiatric symptoms of note. HD genotyping was requested and was negative.

Could Kirsty's movement disorder have been caused by her recent sore throat?

Involuntary, jerky and purposeless movements can occur in some patients following a streptococcal infection. The movements occur sporadically in different muscle groups and in such a manner that the patient is constantly in motion and seems to be twitching everywhere. Fine motor control may become difficult and handwriting may change dramatically. The disorder occurs most frequently in adolescent girls but may be seen in boys.

What diagnostic tests would you request?

Blood tests that may show signs of rheumatic fever include erythrocyte sedimentation rate (ESR), C-reactive protein (CRP) and antistreptolysin O titre (ASOT). Other tests related to acute rheumatic fever include an electrocardiogram (ECG) and echocardiogram.

Kirsty's ESR and CRP were within normal limits but her ASOT was significantly elevated. Her ECG and echocardiogram were normal. Kirsty's diagnosis is Sydenham's chorea (St Vitus dance), a movement disorder associated with rheumatic fever.

How should her condition be treated?

Antibiotics are given to assure clearing of the streptococci, the bacteria that cause rheumatic fever. Continuous preventative antibiotics (antibiotic prophylaxis) may be prescribed if there is evidence of cardiac valvular damage placing the patient at risk of infective endocarditis. Supportive care is given as necessary to control symptoms of Sydenham's chorea.

What is Kirsty's prognosis?

Sydenham's chorea usually resolves spontaneously over a course of several months.

Kirsty's movements gradually settled over the next 3 months and she returned to a full and active life at school. Repeat echocardiography demonstrated no long-term valvular defects in the heart.

CASE REVIEW

This young girl presented with a short history of abnormal choreiform movements developing some time after a probable streptococcal throat infection. All investigations were normal save a strongly positive ASOT, and her condition resolved gradually over a few months, without any evidence of cardiac complications.

KEY POINTS

- Movement disorders often arise from pathology in the basal ganglia or cerebellum
- Movement disorders can be classified as hyperkinesias or hypokinesias
- Akathisia, athetosis, ballismus, chorea, dyskinesia and tremor are all different types of abnormal movements
- Abnormal movements may be caused by drugs including neuroleptics, levodopa, lithium and anticonvulsants
- Causes of chorea include Huntington's disease, hyperthyroidism, pregnancy, the oral contraceptive pill, neuroleptic drugs, SLE and Sydenham's chorea
- Huntington's disease is an autosomal, dominantly inherited disorder that leads to a progressive movement disorder associated with dementia and psychiatric symptoms
- Sydenham's chorea is a post-streptococcal movement disorder. The movement disorder is usually self-limiting and treatment is given with penicillin as the condition is associated with rheumatic fever

Further reading and references

Bhidayasiri R, Truong D. Chorea and related disorders. *Postgrad Med J* 2004;**80**(947):527–34.

Wild EJ, Tabrizi SJ. The differential diagnosis of chorea. *Pract Neurol* 2007;**7**(6):360–73.

MCQs

For each situation, choose the single option you feel is most correct.

> **1** Caroline, a 24-year-old gym instructor, presents with symptoms of a 'pounding' headache over the left side of her head. Headaches occur about once every week and are sometimes preceded by 'dots and blots' in her vision and tingling that starts in her right hand, slowly spreading up her arm. When the headaches come on particularly badly they can last for hours and she often feels very sick. Loud noises are irritating and she finds relief by lying in a dark room.

Which one of the following drug treatments is most effective in treating her acute headache attacks?

A. Propranolol

B. High-flow oxygen

C. Tramadol

D. Soluble aspirin

E. Co-codamol

> **2** Michael Carlisle, a 48-year-old welder, presents with attacks of excruciating pain around his left eye. Episodes of pain begin without warning and reach maximal intensity within 5 minutes. Once the pain has set in, he describes it as 'continuous and explosive' and the discomfort is so bad he has difficulty sitting still. Attacks last from 30 to 90 minutes and are associated with nausea, tearing of his left eye and stuffiness of his nose. His wife has noticed that his left eye is often red during attacks and sometimes also appears droopy. He has had about four attacks a day over the past 3 weeks occurring at around the same time of day. Headaches are often triggered by drinking red wine.

What is the most likely diagnosis in this patient?

A. Migraine

B. Acute angle closure glaucoma

C. An optic nerve tumour

D. Cluster headache

E. Trigeminal neuralgia

> **3** Gregory Adams, a 59-year-old banker, presents to A&E with a severe headache and symptoms of neck stiffness. The headache came on over the back of his head and neck within a matter of seconds earlier that evening shortly after intercourse. He described the pain as 'the worst he has ever experienced' and thinks he may have passed out for a few seconds. He feels very sick and reports having vomited twice. He has a history of hypertension and smokes 20 cigarettes a day. On examination he is alert and orientated and has a GCS of 15. General systemic examination is unremarkable. He has a stiff neck but no focal neurological deficits.

What is the most appropriate next step in this man's management?

A. Perform a lumbar puncture

B. Treat with high-dose intravenous ceftriaxone

C. Reassure the patient that he has experienced a benign coital headache

D. Perform an urgent CT of the head

E. Prescribe 600–900 mg of soluble aspirin

Neurology: Clinical Cases Uncovered, 1st edition. © M. Macleod, M. Simpson and S. Pal. Published 2011 by Blackwell Publishing Ltd.

4 *A 22-year-old woman with epilepsy is contemplating pregnancy.*

Which one of the following statements is true?
A. The risk of serious abnormalities occurring in the fetus is approximately 10 times greater than that of women without epilepsy planning pregnancy
B. Anticonvulsant medications are teratogenic and should, therefore, be stopped in all pregnant women
C. Folic acid should be avoided as this may exacerbate neural tube defects
D. The risk of sudden death in epilepsy is increased if anticonvulsant medication is stopped
E. Anticonvulsant medications have no effect on the oral contraceptive pill

5 *Maureen Brown is a 54-year-old woman with diabetes and a body mass index of 32. She has been waking up at night with uncomfortable pins and needles in both hands and finds that shaking her wrists offers some symptomatic relief.*

What is the most likely diagnosis?
A. Painful ulnar neuropathy
B. Painful radial neuropathy
C. Hyperventilation syndrome
D. Carpal tunnel syndrome
E. Side effects of insulin therapy

6 *Amanda is a 22-year-old who is 12 weeks' pregnant. She has been experiencing troublesome nausea and vomiting for the past 4 weeks and has struggled to keep any food or drink down. She now presents with severe headache and blurring of her vision. She has a past history of a deep vein thrombosis which she attributed to a long haul flight. A detailed family history reveals that her mother has also been treated for 'blood clots in the legs'. On examination, Amanda is slim, her visual acuity is 6/9 on the right and 6/12 on the left. Fundoscopy reveals bilateral blurring of the disc margins.*

What is the most likely diagnosis?
A. Migraine
B. Tension headache
C. Idiopathic intracranial hypertension
D. Intracerebral venous sinus thrombosis
E. Subarachnoid haemorrhage

7 *Albert Webb is an 82-year-old retired civil servant. His past medical history includes hypertension and a previous myocardial infarction. He presents with sudden-onset weakness of his right arm and leg, slurred speech and difficulties expressing himself. On examination his pulse is 84 beats/min and irregular and there is evidence of an ejection systolic murmur. He has evidence of a mixed expressive and receptive dysphasia, a right-sided homonomous hemianopia and dense weakness of his right arm and leg.*

Which one of the following investigations is it most important to conduct next?
A. Coagulation studies (APTT/INR)
B. Carotid Doppler studies
C. Echocardiogram
D. CT head scan
E. Thrombophilia screen

8 *Margaret Hobbs is a 76-year-old lady who presented following sudden-onset weakness of her right face, arm and leg associated with slurred speech and difficulties with expression. She is in sinus rhythm with a blood pressure of 170/90 mmHg. CT and subsequent MRI of the brain confirm an ischaemic stroke affecting the left middle cerebral artery territory.*

In secondary prevention of thromboembolic stroke, which one of the following treatments *has not* been demonstrated to reduce the risk of further stroke in this patient?
A. Warfarin
B. Aspirin
C. Clopidogrel
D. Antihypertensive medication
E. Statin therapy

9 & 10 *Cheryl Bingham is a 27-year-old waitress who presents with ascending numbness, tingling and weakness of her legs leading to difficulties walking. Symptoms seem to have emerged following a diarrhoeal illness 10 days ago and have been worsening such that she now has difficulties standing and walking. On examination she has grade 3–4/5 power in all the muscle groups of both arms and legs with absent reflexes. There is also evidence of distal sensory loss on the upper and lower limbs.*

Which one of the following statements regarding Guillan–Barré syndrome is correct? [Question 9]
A. Cerebrospinal fluid protein is frequently elevated
B. Up to 40% of cases follow an antecedent *Escherichia coli* infection
C Limb reflexes are typically brisk
D. No treatments are effective in hastening recovery
E. Pulmonary complications are rare

Which one of the following statements regarding Guillan–Barré syndrome is true? [Question 10]
A. MRI of the spinal cord demonstrates changes consistent with demyelination
B. Facial weakness is extremely uncommon
C. The diagnosis can be made following MRI of the brain
D. Cardiac arrhythmias and fluctuations in blood pressure are a recognised complication
E. Nerve conduction studies are only rarely useful

11 *Colin Archer is a 53-year-old man who attends the A&E department following a deliberate overdose of paracetamol and sleeping tablets. He reports low mood, loss of interest in his usual hobbies, poor sleep and generally feeling that 'life is not worth living anymore'. Neurological examination reveals some extrapyramidal signs and review of his medical records reveals that he is under review in the neurology clinic.*

Which one of the following movement disorders is associated with the highest risk of depression and suicidal ideation?
A. Wilson's disease
B. Parkinson's disease
C. Multiple system atrophy
D. Huntington's disease
E. Corticobasal degeneration

12 *Andrew Dewar is an 82-year-old man who presents with a history of increasing confusion over the past 4 months associated with gait dyspraxia and urinary incontinence. A CT brain scan demonstrates enlargement of the lateral ventricles but not the cerebral sulci.*

Which one of the following is the most likely diagnosis?
A. Parkinson's disease
B. Progressive supranuclear gaze palsy
C. Alzheimer's disease
D. Normal pressure hydrocephalus
E. Dementia with Lewy bodies

13 & 14 *Andy Carter is a 35-year-old man who presents with symptoms of double vision and droopiness of both eyelids which he first noticed several weeks ago. More recently he has also noticed heaviness of his legs and arms with particular difficulties climbing up several flights of stairs. His symptoms seem to get worse as the day goes on and are much worse in the evenings. On examination he has evidence of bilateral partial ptosis, worse on the left, and experiences double vision in all directions of gaze. When testing power, shoulder abduction and hip flexion can be overcome and his weakness deteriorates after exercise.*

Which one of the following tests is most likely to provide the diagnosis? [Question 13]
A. Antivoltage gated calcium channel antibody
B. Antivoltage gated potassium channel antibody
C. Antineuronal antibodies
D. Anti-acetylcholine receptor antibody
E. Antiganglioside antibody

Which one of the following treatments is most likely to provide symptomatic benefit? [Question 14]
A. Sodium valproate
B. Pyridostigmine
C. Beta-interferon
D. Riluzole
E. Vitamin B12 replacement

15 & 16 *Philip Noble, a 72-year-old retired dentist, presents with pain around his jaw after chewing. He has also been experiencing headaches above his right eye and on examination has some tenderness over his right temple.*

Which one of the following is the most appropriate next investigation? [Question 15]
A. Cerebrospinal fluid examination to measure the opening pressure
B. CT brain scan
C. Serum erythrocyte sedimentation rate (ESR)
D. X-ray of the mandibles
E. Dental X-rays

Which one of the following treatments is most appropriate? [Question 16]
A. Relaxation strategies
B. A ventriculoperitoneal shunt
C. High-dose oral steroids (1 mg/kg)
D. Tooth extraction
E. Regular co-codamol

17 *Mary Black is a 56-year-old music teacher who complains of unsteadiness whilst walking. She also has symptoms of constipation and difficulties passing water. There is no past medical history of note and she takes no regular medications. On examination her blood pressure is 140/96 mmHg lying and 90/64 mmHg standing. She walks with short shuffling steps and has evidence of bradykinesia and tremulousness of her hands.*

Which of the following is her most likely diagnosis?
A. Benign essential tremor
B. Idiopathic Parkinson's disease
C. Normal pressure hydrocephalus
D. Dementia with Lewy bodies
E. Multiple system atrophy

18 *Alfred Baxter is a 62-year-old joiner who complains of double vision when he looks to his left. He has a background of type 2 diabetes which is poorly controlled. Alfred does not check his blood glucose very often but when he does levels vary between 9 and 19 mmol/L. A recent HbA1c was 12%. On examination he experiences double vision when pursuing an object with horizontal separation of images. The double vision is worst with maximal separation of images on looking to the left. When he covers the left eye, the outermost image disappears.*

Which one of the following cranial nerves is most likely to be affected?
A. Left oculomotor nerve
B. Right oculomotor nerve
C. Left optic nerve
D. Left trochlear nerve
E. Left abducens nerve

19 *David Elliot is a 45-year-old journalist who presents with symptoms of progressive deafness in his right ear for the past year. Over the past few weeks he has noticed that he is unsteady on his feet and veers off to the right when he walks. On examination there is evidence of nystagmus on horizontal gaze to the right. The right corneal reflex is absent and his hearing is reduced on the right.*

Which one of the following is the most likely diagnosis?
A. Multiple sclerosis
B. A brainstem stroke
C. An acoustic neuroma
D. Meniere's disease
E. Malignant otitis externa

20 *Marie Jennings is a 19-year-old vet student who presents to A&E at 8 pm following a 2-day history of high fevers, headache and vomiting. On examination her temperature is 38°C and her pulse is 128 beats/min with a blood pressure of 96/68 mmHg. She is disorientated and there is evidence of a petechial rash extending over her trunk and arms. She is photophobic with neck stiffness and Kernig's sign is positive.*

Which one of the following is the most appropriate next step in her management?
A. Lumbar puncture
B. MRI brain scan
C. Blood cultures followed by high-dose intravenous antibiotics
D. Intubation and transfer to the intensive care unit
E. Urgent neurosurgical review

21 & 22 *Gwyneth McAndrew is a 34-year-old female who presents with abnormal involuntary choreiform movements and cognitive decline which has progressed over the past few years. Her father committed suicide at the age of 46. On examination her Mini-Mental State Examination score is 18 out of 30. She has continuous choreiform movements of her hands and feet. Power is preserved in all muscle groups and all of her reflexes are present. She has no cerebellar signs and sensory examination is normal.*

Which of the following is the most likely diagnosis? [Question 21]
A. Juvenile Parkinson's disease
B. Wilson's disease
C. Sporadic Creutzfeldt–Jakob disease
D. Huntington's disease
E. Multiple sclerosis

Which one of the following statements is true regarding Gwyneth's illness? [Question 22]
A. Her condition is inherited in an autosomal recessive manner
B. Her condition is inherited in an autosomal dominant manner
C. Her condition is X-linked
D. The diagnosis can be achieved by analysis of cerebrospinal fluid
E. The diagnosis can only be clear after a brain biopsy or at postmortem

23 *Mabel Rogers is a 78-year-old woman who presents to clinic accompanied by her daughter Kate. Kate is concerned about her mother's memory. Over the last few months she has been missing appointments and has been increasingly forgetful about contents of recent conversations. She has been struggling with complex tasks at home such as cooking and, on one occasion recently, Mabel got lost on her way back from the shops on a route that is very familiar to her. Mabel has been struggling with things at home recently and almost had her electricity and gas supplies cut off as she forgot to pay her bills. Mable's past medical history includes osteoporosis. On examination, Mabel has difficulties with short-term recall whilst memory for remote events appeared preserved. Her Mini-Mental State Examination score was 23/30. The remainder of the neurological examination was grossly unremarkable.*

Which one of the following is the most likely diagnosis?
A. Dementia with Lewy bodies
B. Vascular dementia
C. Alzheimer's disease
D. Depression
E. Transient global amnesia

24 *Shona King is a 26-year-old driving instructor with myasthenia gravis. She presents to A&E with a chest infection which has resulted in decreased exercise tolerance, breathlessness, slurred speech and some difficulties with swallowing.*

Which one of the following is the most reliable measure of respiratory function in patients with severe neuromuscular weakness?
A. Peak expiratory flow rate
B. Peripheral oxygen saturation
C. Arterial blood gas measurement
D. Vital capacity
E. Patient's ability to speak in full sentences

25 Adman Chilcott is a 48-year-old music teacher with a 2-day history of headache, fever and worsening confusion who is taken by ambulance to A&E following a generalised tonic-clonic seizure. On examination his temperature is 38°C and he is confused with expressive dysphasia. Viral encephalitis is suspected.

Which one of the following statements regarding viral encephalitis is true?

A. Treatment should only be started after a virus has been isolated from the cerebrospinal fluid
B. MRI of the brain is usually normal
C. A travel history is rarely of relevance
D. In herpes simplex encephalitis stereotyped sharp and slow complexes may be seen on an EEG originating from the temporal lobes
E. Brain biopsy remains the primary diagnostic test for viral encephalits

26 Margaret Adamson is a 53-year-old librarian who presents with episodic attacks of excruciating pain affecting the lips, and cheek over the right side of her face. Episodes are triggered by touching her face over the affected areas, and even by cold wind blowing on the face. Neurological examination is entirely normal.

What is the most likely diagnosis?

A. Multiple sclerosis
B. Temporal arteritis
C. Trigeminal neuralgia
D. Cluster headache
E. Facial nerve palsy

27 John Wilkinson is a 18-year-old A level student who presents with episode of 'odd behaviour'. Over the past 2 weeks he has had three episodes witnessed by his friends and teachers during which he stares ahead blankly. Prior to one of these episodes, John remembers a strong smell of oranges. Moments after experiencing the smell, John appeared vacant and was unable to respond to people around him. Each episode lasted around 30 seconds and his eyes were always open. Just afterwards he made 'odd chewing movements' and 'smacked his lips' for around 20 seconds. He remained confused for about an hour after each episode and afterwards had no recollection for the events he experienced.

Which one of the following is the most likely diagnosis?

A. Syncopal episodes
B. Absence seizures
C. Complex partial seizure
D. Generalised tonic clonic (grand mal) seizure
E. Narcolepsy

28 Sarah Horner presents to the first seizure clinic following a history of episodes consistent with generalised tonic-clonic seizures.

Which one of the following statements regarding epilepsy is true?

A. Patients presenting following a first seizure should be advised to surrender their driving licence and stop driving indefinitely
B. Patients with epilepsy must remain on anticonvulsant medications for life
C. The incidence of depression and suicide is no greater in patients with epilepsy than in the general population
D. Patients with epilepsy should be warned there is a risk of sudden unexpected death associated with their illness
E. Acute infections are the commonest cause of seizures in the elderly

29 Alfred Sharpe is a 50-year-old an who presents following a 6-month history of weakness affecting his arms and legs. On examination there is evidence of widespread muscle wasting with fasiculations, particularly over his thighs. Tone is increased in the legs and reflexes are brisk throughout. Motor neuron disease is suspected.

Which one of the following statements is true regarding motor neuron disease?

A. Most cases are inherited in an autosomal dominant manner
B. The diagnosis is achieved by analysis of cerebrospinal fluid
C. Riluzole reverses neurological symptoms in the majority of patients
D. The main cause of death is related to respiratory failure and chest infections
E. Sensory symptoms are common

30 *Ella Shand is a 24-year-old receptionist who presents following an episode of painful visual loss 1 year ago and more recent progressive weakness of her left leg, worsening over the past 3 weeks. Her GP has referred her to the neurology clinic worried she may have multiple sclerosis.*

Which one of the following statements is true regarding multiple sclerosis?

A. Beta-interferon has been demonstrated to successfully cure the majority of patients with the illness

B. Vision is only rarely affected in the condition

C. All patients presenting with a deterioration in neurological symptoms should be offered high-dose intravenous steroids

D. The presence of oligoclonal bands in the serum supports a diagnosis of this condition

E. Optic neuritis is the presenting symptom in approximately 40% of patients diagnosed with this

EMQs

1 Cranial nerves

A. CN III (oculomotor)
B. CN IV (trochlear)
C. CN V (trigeminal)
D. CN VI (abducens)
E. CN VII (facial)
F. CN XI (accessory)

Match the following muscles with the corresponding cranial nerves from the list above:

1. Inferior rectus
2. Sternocleidomastoid
3. Orbicularis oculi
4. Masseter
5. Inferior oblique
6. Trapezius
7. Lateral rectus
8. Frontalis
9. Medial rectus
10. Superior oblique

2 Dermatomes

A. C4
B. C5
C. C6
D. C7
E. C8
F. T1
G. T5
H. T10
I. L5
J. S1

Match the following areas of the body with their corresponding dermatome (sensory nerve root), listed above:

1. Lateral aspect of the upper arms
2. Medial aspect of the lower arms
3. Tip of the thumb
4. Sole of the foot
5. Tip of the middle finger
6. Posterior aspect of the shoulders
7. Tip of the little finger
8. Nipple
9. Lateral aspect of the lower leg
10. Umbilicus

Neurology: Clinical Cases Uncovered, 1st edition. © M. Macleod, M. Simpson and S. Pal. Published 2011 by Blackwell Publishing Ltd.

PART 3: SELF-ASSESSMENT

3 Nerve functions

A. Facial sensation, movements of the jaw and corneal reflexes
B. Hearing and balance
C. Smell
D. Facial movements and taste to the anterior two-thirds of the tongue
E. Tongue movements
F. Visual acuity, visual fields and ocular fundi
G. Abduction of the eye
H. Adduction and vertical movements of the eye
I. Sensation of the posterior pharyngeal wall, gag reflex and taste to the posterior two-thirds of the tongue
J. Shrugging the shoulders and turning the head
K. Depression, intorsion and abduction of the eye
L. Autonomic supply to the thoracic and abdominal viscera, and elevation of the palate

Match the following cranial nerves with their corresponding function, listed above:

1. I, olfactory
2. II, optic
3. III, oculomotor
4. IV, trochlear
5. V, trigeminal
6. VI, abducens
7. VII, facial
8. VIII, vestibulocochlear
9. IX, glossopharyngeal
10. X, vagus
11. XI, accessory
12. XII, hypoglossal

4 Nerve roots

A. S1 nerve root
B. C5 and C6 nerve roots
C. C6 and C7 nerve roots, predominantly C7
D. Trigeminal nerve root
E. L3 and L4 nerve roots, mainly L4

Match the following reflexes with their corresponding nerve roots (above):

1. Jaw jerk
2. Ankle Jerk
3. Biceps reflex
4. Triceps reflex
5. Knee jerk
6. Brachioradialis reflex

5 Neurological diagnosis

A. Herpes simplex encephalitis
B. Bacterial meningitis
C. Idiopathic seizures
D. Subarachnoid haemorrhage
E. Multiple sclerosis

Match the following cerebrospinal fluid findings with the most likely neurological diagnosis:

1. Clear CSF with normal opening pressure, normal protein, normal glucose, and no white or red blood cells
2. Cloudy CSF with mildly elevated opening pressure, increased protein, decreased glucose, and high white blood cells (predominately polymorphs)
3. Pink/yellow CSF with increased opening pressure, elevated, protein, normal glucose, slightly elevated white blood cells, and significantly elevated red cells
4. Cloudy CSF with increased opening pressure, elevated protein, normal glucose, increased white blood cells (predominantly lymphocytes), and a few red blood cells
5. Clear CSF with normal opening pressure, mildly elevated protein, normal glucose, a few white blood cells (predominantly lymphocytes), no red blood cells, and positive oligoclonal bands.

6 Drugs

A. Levodopa
B. Sodium valproate
C. Propranolol
D. Pyridostigmine
E. Prednisolone
F. Intravenous immunoglobulin

Match the patient diagnosis with the correct pharmacological therapy (one or more of the drugs listed above may be correct):

1. Myasthenia gravis
2. Parkinson's disease
3. Generalised seizures
4. Frequent migraine
5. Essential tremor
6. Guillan–Barré syndrome
7. Temporal arteritis

7 Investigations
A. Lumbar puncture
B. Nerve conduction studies
C. MRI brain scan
D. Molecular diagnostic testing
E. Acetylcholine receptor antibody
F. Electroencephalogram
G. Full blood count
H. Vitamin B12 levels
I. MRI of the spine
J. Creatinine phosphokinase levels
K. Muscle biopsy
L. CT head scan

Match the following conditions with the investigations that are most useful in their diagnosis (one or more of the above may apply):
1. Subarachnoid haemorrhage
2. Motor neuron disease
3. Dermatomyositis
4. Myasthenia gravis
5. Multiple sclerosis
6. Viral encephalitis
7. Subacute combined degeneration of the cord
8. Alcohol-induced neuropathy
9. Myotonic dystrophy

8 Lesion site
A. Temporal lobe
B. Optic chiasm
C. Occipital lobe
D. Parietal lobe
E. Retina

Match the following visual field defects by the site of lesion:
1. Inferior quadrantic hemianopia
2. Congruous hemianopia with macular sparing
3. Bitemporal hemianopia
4. Inferior quadrantic hemianopia
5. Monocular blindness

9 Site of peripheral nerve lesion
A. Median nerve
B. Ulnar nerve
C. Common peroneal nerve
D. Lateral cutaneous nerve of the thigh
E. Radial nerve

Match the corresponding symptoms and signs with the corresponding peripheral nerve lesion listed above:
1. An area of numbness and burning on the outer aspect of the thigh
2. Numbness and tingling of the little and ring finger; weakness and wasting of the dorsal interossei and abductor digiti minimi; sensory disturbance over the little and ring fingers
3. Weakness of the wrist and finger extensors; sensory numbness over the dorsal surface of the hand near the base of the thumb
4. 'Foot drop' with weakness of ankle dorsiflexion, toe extension and foot eversion with preservation of foot inversion; sensory loss over the lateral aspect of the foot and calf
5. Numbness and tingling of the hand, waking patients from sleep; weakness and, sometimes, wasting of the abductor pollicis brevis; sensory disturbance over the lateral three and a half digits; positive Tinel's and Phalen's signs

> **10 Diagnosis**
> **A.** Headache of raised intracranial pressure
> **B.** Migraine
> **C.** Trigeminal neuralgia
> **D.** Temporal arteritis
> **E.** Subarachnoid haemorrhage

Match the following clinical vignettes with the correct diagnosis:

1. Episodes of sudden severe stabbing pain in a 48-year-old man occurring over the face and lasting from seconds to minutes. The pain occurs in bouts occurring up to several times a day and can be triggered by touch

2. A sudden-onset, severe occipital headache reaching maximal intensity within seconds and associated with nausea and vomiting in a 59-year-old man with a past history of hypertension and smoking

3. A 28-year-old woman with a right-sided frontal throbbing headache associated with dots and blots in her vision, nausea, photophobia and a tingling of the right hand

4. A pain over the temples in a 72-year-old woman associated with visual blurring, worsening pain on chewing and combing the hair, anorexia and weight loss

5. A dull frontal headache in a 24-year-old man that is worse in the morning and on bending forwards, coughing and sneezing. There is associated nausea, vomiting and blurring of vision

SAQs

1 *A 73-year-old man with a background of hypertension and atrial fibrillation presents following a fall 1 week ago and symptoms of a headache with unsteadiness on walking. On examination he has papilloedema with brisk reflexes and an upgoing left plantar response.*

A. What would you be concerned about from this history?
B. What investigations would you organise?
C. A CT head was obtained (Fig. S1.1): what does this show?
D. How should this man be treated?

2 *Karen Roberts is a 32-year-old nurse who presents following 2 weeks of early morning headache, visual blurring and numbness of her left hand. The headache is worse when she coughs, sneezes or strains on stool. On examination, there is evidence of a left superior quadrantinopia, hyperreflexia and upgoing plantars bilaterally.*

A. What would you be concerned about from this history?
B. Which area of the brain does the visual field defect localise the lesion to?
C. What investigation would you arrange?
D. What does the CT with contrast of the head (Fig. S2.1) reveal?
E. What treatment may help with symptoms in the short term?
F. What imaging would you arrange next?
G. What does the T2-weighted MRI of the brain (Fig. S2.2) show?

H. What other tests may be performed?
I. What are the general options available for the treatment of primary brain tumours?

3 *Jack Alexander, a 68-year-old farmer, presents to the neurology clinic with his wife. Mrs Alexander reports that Jack has been more irritable over the past 6 months and has become increasingly forgetful, often missing appointments, losing personal items and having difficulties remembering the content of recent conversations. More recently, he has accused his neighbours of continuously watching his house and is now reluctant to go outdoors alone. His GP recently prescribed flupentixol tablets to help him relax. On examination, his blood pressure was 148/78 mmHg lying and 112/72 mmHg standing. Bedside cognitive tests demonstrated a Mini mental State Examination score of 18 out of 30 with deficits in orientation, concentration and recall. Facial expression was reduced. Examination of eye movements demonstrated a mild limitation of upgaze. Tone was increased in the limbs with symmetrical reflexes and bilateral downgoing plantars. There was impairment of rapid alternating finger movements and evidence of micrographia. Gait demonstrated shuffling steps with reduced arm swing.*

A. What is the most likely diagnosis?
B. What is the differential diagnosis?
C. What intervention may improve his current symptoms?

Neurology: Clinical Cases Uncovered, 1st edition. © M. Macleod, M. Simpson and S. Pal. Published 2011 by Blackwell Publishing Ltd.

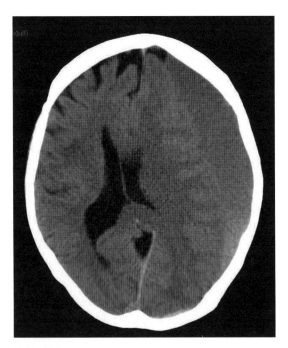

Figure S1.1

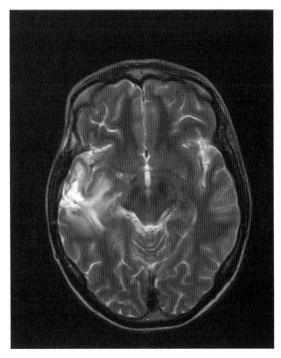

Figure S2.2

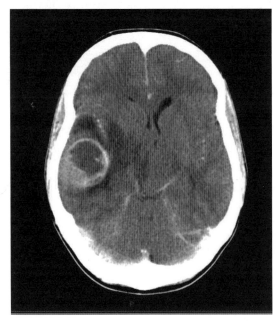

Figure S2.1

4 *A 53-year-old man is referred by his general practitioner with a tremor affecting his left wrist and hand. This has been present for the past 8 months and is present intermittently but seems to worsen with stress or anxiety. He also reports feeling generally fatigued and low in mood. He has noticed a subtle decrease in dexterity and lack of coordination with activities such as playing golf. On examination he is noted to have a simple oscillating tremor of the left hand, which is present at rest. The same tremor is noticed with the arms outstretched. Assessment of tone reveals cogwheeling in the distal left upper limb. Examination of his gait reveals small steps with reduced arm swing of the left upper limb and postural instability on tests of retropulsion.*

A. What is the most likely diagnosis?
B. What are the characteristics of tremor in this disease?
C. What treatment strategies are available?

5 *A 68-year-old librarian complains of clumsiness of his left hand with deterioration in handwriting. His symptoms have been present for the last 3 months and began after an influenza-like illness. More recently he has experienced a sensation of the 'world spinning around'. Cranial nerve examination reveals nystagmus on left lateral gaze with diminished sensation over the left side of the face and an absent left corneal reflex. On examination of the limbs, there is impairment of finger–nose coordination in the left upper limb with impaired rapid alternating movement of the hands.*

A. What is the next investigation of choice?
B. What does the MRI of the brain (Fig. S5.1) show?
C. What is the most likely diagnosis?
D. What other lesions may arise at this anatomical location?
E. Which cranial nerve is involved clinically in this case?
F. What other cranial nerves may be involved with a lesion at the cerebellopontine angle?
G. What diagnosis should be considered if bilateral vestibular schwannomas are present?

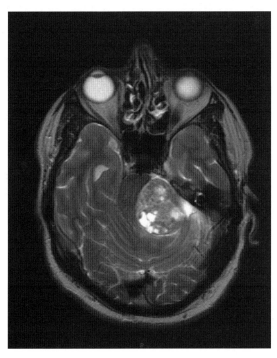

Figure S5.1

6 *Asif, an 18-year-old man from Saudia Arabia, has been referred by the psychiatrists for advice after the following blood test results were obtained:*

Hb	10.2 g/dL
WCC	9.3 × 10⁹/L
Platelets	290 × 10⁹/L
MCV	103 fL
Sodium	138 mmol/L
Potassium	4.8 mmol/L
Urea	3.9 mmol/L
Creatinine	70 μmol/L
Bilirubin	40 μmol/L
Albumin	29 g/L
GGT	120 IU/L
AST	80 IU/L
ALP	270 IU/L

A collateral history from Asif's parents suggests that his personality has changed over the past year in that he has become hostile and irritable. His A level grades were significantly worse than anticipated and his teachers have commented that he has been unusually unruly during lessons. On examination there is evidence of hepatosplenomegaly. His Mini-Mental State Examination score is 25/30. He has a mild slurring dysarthria and a tremor affecting his right upper limb. Rapid alternating movements of the fingers were slow. A detailed family history reveals that Asif has a maternal uncle and two cousins with a variety of neurological symptoms although no firm diagnosis has been achieved.

A. What is the most likely diagnosis?
B. What is the mode of inheritance of this condition?
C. What diagnostic sign may be present in the eyes?
D. What other tests are useful diagnostically?
E. How is this condition treated?

7 *A 49-year-old barrister is referred to the outpatient clinic for further investigation of troublesome headaches. He reports attacks of very severe burning pain. The pain develops over a few minutes on the left side of his head behind the eye. Sometimes he feels nauseous and occasionally notices the pain spreading to his forehead. Attacks last from 20 minutes to an hour and occur up to three times a day. The attacks are frequently associated with a runny nose. His wife reports that he often paces about banging his head with his fist during episodes and seems tearful. He mentions that he feels under particular stress at work with recent difficulties meeting deadlines for preparing lectures and marking coursework. He often lies in bed worrying about his symptoms and has lost his appetite. His younger sister suffers from migraines and his mother is on medication for depression. He drinks about 5 pints of beer at weekends although has reduced this recently as he feels it aggravates the headaches.*

A. What is the most likely diagnosis?
B. What is the typical duration of such attacks?
C. Which site of the head is usually affected?
D. What associated features may be present?
E. What is the character of pain in this type of headache?
F. What treatments may abort such attacks?
G. Which prophylactic treatments are considered effective?
H. What are the surgical management options?

8 *A 71-year-old engineer was reviewed in the outpatient clinic with symptoms of weakness in his arms and 'twitching' of his thighs. His difficulties started 3 months ago when he noticed difficulties shelving heavy objects in his garage at home. Three weeks ago he noticed weakness affecting his left hand. His family has noticed that his speech has become slurred and that he is uncharacteristically tearful. He has lost 8 kg of weight in the past year. He has smoked 10 cigarettes a day for the past 25 years and drinks 5 pints of ale a week. Cranial nerve examination was unremarkable. Fasiculations were noted over both scapular regions with wasting of the small muscles of the left hand. Power was reduced in all muscle groups of the left upper limb. Examination of the lower limbs demonstrated fasiculations over the quadriceps bilaterally with difficulty rising from a low chair. Reflexes were symmetrically brisk with bilateral upgoing plantars. Sensory examination was normal.*

A. What is the most likely diagnosis in this case?
B. What is the differential diagnosis?
C. Which investigations are useful diagnostically?
D. Who else would you involve in the patient's management?
E. What feeding options are present if swallowing is deemed unsafe?

9 *A 38-year-old woman presents following a sudden-onset headache. She describes the pain as the worst she has ever experienced and that it came on within seconds over the back of her head. The headache is associated with nausea and vomiting. Her neck is stiff and bright lights are sore. On examination she is alert and orientated with no focal neurological deficits.*

A. What diagnosis must be excluded?
B. What risk factors predispose to this condition?
C. What is the investigation of choice?
D. What does this patient's CT of the head (Fig. S9.1) demonstrate?
E. What further investigations are indicated?
F. What is the treatment of choice?
G. What are the main immediate complications?

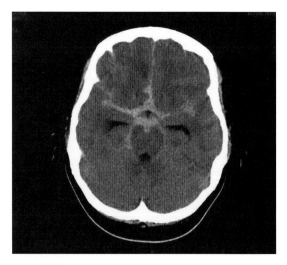

Figure S9.1

10 A 46-year-old man presents with weakness in his hands and legs. In particular he reports difficulties playing football with his sons. On examination he has evidence of a bilateral ptosis. Fundoscopy proves difficult because of bilateral cataracts. Facial expression is reduced with wasting of the temporalis muscles, masseters and sternomastoids. You notice a slow release of hand grip bilaterally after shaking his hands, with weakness and wasting in the distal muscles of the upper limb.

A. What is the most likely diagnosis in this case?
B. What are the systemic complications of this disease?
C. What is the underlying aetiology of this condition?
D. What do you understand by the phenomenon of genetic anticipation?
E. Which diagnostic tests are of use?

MCQ answers

1. D	11. D	21. D
2. D	12. D	22. B
3. D	13. D	23. C
4. D	14. B	24. D
5. D	15. C	25. D
6. D	16. C	26. C
7. D	17. E	27. C
8. A	18. E	28. D
9. A	19. C	29. D
10. D	20. C	30. E

Neurology: Clinical Cases Uncovered, 1st edition. © M. Macleod,
M. Simpson and S. Pal. Published 2011 by Blackwell Publishing Ltd.

EMQ answers

1
1. A
2. F
3. E
4. C
5. A
6. F
7. D
8. E
9. A
10. B

2
1. B
2. F
3. C
4. J
5. D
6. A
7. E
8. G
9. I
10. H

3
1. C
2. F
3. H
4. K
5. A
6. G
7. D
8. B
9. I

10. L
11. J
12. E

4
1. D
2. A
3. B
4. C
5. E
6. B

5
1. C
2. B
3. D
4. A
5. E

6
1. D, E, F
2. A
3. B
4. C, B
5. C
6. F
7. E

7
1. L, A
2. B
3. J, B, K
4. E, B
5. C, A, I

6. A, C, F
7. H, I
8. G, B
9. D, B

8
1. A
2. C
3. B
4. D
5. E

9
1. D
2. B
3. E
4. C
5. A

10
1. C
2. E
3. B
4. D
5. A

PART 3: SELF-ASSESSMENT

1

A. The history suggests new neurological symptoms that have emerged following trauma. The examination findings include upper motor neuron signs suggestive of a space-occupying lesion.

B. Routine blood tests demonstrated normal results and an INR of 3.8.

C. There is a large, acute or chronic, left *subdural haematoma* which is causing a considerable mass effect with displacement of the left lateral ventricle and significant midline shift.

D. The deranged INR is most probably secondary to warfarin therapy for atrial fibrillation. This should be corrected. In view of the significant mass effect, this man should be referred to neurosurgeons for assessment of surgical evacuation of the haematoma.

2

A. The features are suggestive of a raised intracranial pressure headache with upper motor neuron signs suggestive of a space-occupying lesion.

B. The right temporal lobe

C. Neuroimaging; in the first instance, CT is usually more readily available than MRI.

D. There is a rim-enhancing mass lesion in the right temporal lobe. This has a hyperdense periphery that shows contrast enhancement indicating marked surrounding oedema and localised mass effect. The temporal horn of the right lateral ventricle is displaced medially and there is almost complete effacement of the right lateral ventricle and midline shift. The appearances are consistent with a primary cerebral tumour although a solitary metastatic or an abcess are also possibilities.

Neurology: Clinical Cases Uncovered, 1st edition. © M. Macleod,
M. Simpson and S. Pal. Published 2011 by Blackwell Publishing Ltd.

E. Steroids (in the form of intravenous or oral dexamethasone) may help to reduce oedema and mass effect around the tumour and may lead to a transient improvement of symptoms.

F. MRI of the brain is the next most appropriate step to delineate the lesion further. If a cerebral metastasis is suspected, a thorough systemic examination for lymphadenopathy and masses should be performed together with a chest X-ray and CT of the chest, abdomen and pelvis.

G. As with the CT scan, an abnormality is seen in the right temporal lobe with surrounding oedema. The appearances are likely to represent a primary brain tumour.

H. A brain biopsy was conducted which provided histological confirmation of a high-grade glioma.

I. Depending on the site of the tumour, and histological grade at biopsy, tumours may be amenable to surgical resection or debulking, radiotherapy and chemotherapy. In many cases, however, the prognosis remains poor despite these options and palliative approaches may need to be employed.

3

A. The clinical scenario is suggestive of diffuse Lewy body dementia. This condition is characterised by cognitive impairment with extrapyramidal symptoms. Visual hallucinations and paranoid ideation may be present.

B. The differential diagnosis in this case includes idiopathic Parkinson's disease, multiple system atrophy, progresssive supranuclear palsy and lead poisoning. The diagnosis can only be confirmed by postmortem examination or cortical brain biopsy in life.

C. Extrapyramidal side effects are the most troublesome side effect of the phenothiazine antipsychotics. Flupentixol is likely to have exacerbated symptoms and should be stopped in this case. Parkinsonian symptoms, dystonia, dyskinesia, akathisia and tardive dyskinesia cannot be predicted accurately because they depend on dose and individual susceptibility.

4

A. The clinical scenario is suggestive of Parkinson's disease (PD). Over time, patients notice symptoms related to progressive tremor, bradykinesia, rigidity and gait difficulty. Other initial symptoms of PD may be non-specific and include fatigue and depression. The three cardinal signs of PD are resting tremor, rigidity and bradykinesia. Of these cardinal features, two of three are required to make the clinical diagnosis.

B. The onset of Parkinsonian symptoms is typically asymmetrical, with the most common initial finding being resting tremor in an upper extremity. The tremor tends to be present at rest at a frequency of 4–6 Hz with a 'pill rolling' character.

C. Dopamine replacement strategies include dopamine agonists and levodopa preparations. Other treatments used include monoamine oxidase B inhibitors, catechol-methyltransferase inhibitors and amantadine. The goal of medical management of PD is to provide control of signs and symptoms for as long as possible while minimising adverse effects. Medications usually provide good symptomatic control for 4–6 years. After this, disability progresses despite best medical management, and many patients develop long-term motor complications including fluctuations and dyskinesia. The younger the patient, the more emphasis is placed on long-term considerations to guide early treatment. Young patients have a longer life expectancy and are more likely to develop motor fluctuations and dyskinesia. For older patients, less emphasis is placed on long-term considerations; the focus is on providing adequate symptomatic benefit in the near term with as few adverse effects as possible.

5

A. Neuroimaging, preferably MRI of the brain.

B. There is a solid and cystic extra-axial mass centred at the left cerebellopontine angle, which compresses the 4th ventricle and pons and causes supratentorial hydrocephalus.

C. The appearances are of a left vestibular schwannoma (acoustic neuroma).

D. Other space-occupying lesions include a cerebellopontine angle glioma and cerebellopontine angle meningioma.

E. Diminshed facial sensation and an absent corneal reflex suggest involvement of the left trigeminal nerve.

F. Deficits may also be apparant in the abducens (VI), facial (VII) and vestibulocochlear (VIII) nerves.

G. Bilateral vestibular schwannoma (acoustic neuromas) are found in neurofibramatosis type 2 (the gene for which is on the long arm of chromosome 22).

6

A. He has evidence of macroytic anaemia with deranged liver function tests. The deranged liver function tests in association with behavioural symptoms, hepatosplenomegaly, cognitive impairment and neurological signs are suggestive of *Wilson's disease*. Liver cirrhosis may arise in addition to movement disorders such as orofacial rigidity, Parkinsonism, tremor and dystonia.

B. The inheritance is autosomal recessive.

C. *Kayser–Fleisher rings* may occur although slit lamp examination may be required for their visualisation.

D. Hepatic biopsy may demonstrate hepatitis and cirrhosis with increased copper content. Measurement of free serum copper, total serum copper, serum caeruloplasmin and 24-hour urinary copper are also diagnostic.

E. Copper chelators, penicillamine and triamterene are often used with varying degrees of success.

7

A. The clinical scenario is suggestive of cluster headaches.

B. Attacks of cluster headaches are typically short in duration (5–180 minutes) and occur with a frequency from once every other day to eight times a day, particularly during sleep.

C. Pain is typically periorbital but may radiate to the face and neck.

D. The association of prominent autonomic phenomena is one of the hallmarks of cluster headache. Signs include ipsilateral nasal congestion and rhinorrhoea, lacrimation, conjunctival hyperaemia, palpebral oedema and complete or partial Horner's syndrome (which may persist between attacks).

E. Pain is generally described as 'excruciating' or 'penetrating', and not 'throbbing' as in migraine. Men are affected more commonly and attacks may result in patients becoming extremely restless, often rocking, pacing around or banging their heads.

F. Inhalation of high-flow concentrated oxygen is an extremely effective therapy for aborting a cluster headache attack. Other strategies include subcutaneous sumitriptan.

G. Effective prophylactic therapy is considered the cornerstone of treatment. Calcium channel blockers inhibit the initial vasoconstrictive phase of cluster headache. Verapamil is perhaps most effective calcium channel blocker for prophylaxis.

H. Invasive nerve blocks and ablative neurosurgical procedures (such as percutaneous radiofrequency, trigeminal gangliorhizolysis and rhizotomy) have been implemented successfully in refractory cases. More recently, gamma-knife radiosurgery has provided a less invasive alternative for pervasive cluster headache.

8

A. The symptoms and signs suggest a progressive degenerative process. The mixture of upper (brisk reflexes with upgoing plantars) and lower (muscle wasting and fasiculations) motor neuron signs suggests anterior horn cell disease. Motor neuron disease presents with proximal or distal asymmetrical weakness of the limbs, or with bulbar dysfunction. Deficits are often accompanied by leg cramps and fasiculation in the proximal limb muscles.

B. The differential diagnosis includes pathology in the brainstem leading to difficulties with speech and swallowing and consequent weight loss, a cervical myelopathy secondary to spondylosis and degenerative disease, and a paranoplastic process with progressive weight loss.

C. Nerve conduction studies and electromyography are helpful in establishing the diagnosis, however the overall diagnosis remains clinical. Imaging of the brain and cervical cord is important in excluding an underlying inflammatory process and cervical myelopathy. A lumbar puncture is useful for excluding an inflammatory or malignant process. CT of the chest, abdomen and pelvis, and antineuronal antibodies, may help in excluding a paraneoplastic process.

D. A speech and language therapy assessment is crucial. Communication may be improved by use of electronic aids. A video fluoroscopy may help investigate dysphagia and risk of aspiration. Physiotherapists and occupational therapists are able to provide practical support with mobility and aids at home.

E. A radiologically or percutaneously inserted gastrostomy (RIG/PEG) tube may be inserted in order to maintain adequate nutrition in cases where swallowing is unsafe.

9

A. The history of sudden-onset headache with maximal intensity within seconds is highly suggestive of a subarachnoid haemorrhage.

B. Hypertension, cigarette smoking, alcohol excess and a history of subarachnoid haemorrhage in more than one first-degree relative are all risk factors for subarachnoid haemorrhage. There is also an association with polycystic kidneys and connective tissue disorders.

C. The investigation of choice is a plain CT of the head. If this is normal, a lumbar puncture should be done looking for xanthochromia and spectroscopy for oxyhaemoglobin and bilirubin.

D. There is evidence of extensive subarachnoid blood. Blood can be seen tracking into the interhemispheric fissure, Sylvian fissures bilaterally, the entire suprasellar cistern and interpeduncular cisterns. There is obvious sulci effacement and dilation of the temporal horns in keeping with raised intracranial pressure. The appearances are in keeping with an acute subarachnoid haemorrhage.

E. A CT angiogram (or formal catheter angiogram) is indicated to investigate for the presence of underlying cerebral aneurysms.

F. Wherever possible, patients with aneurysmal subarachnoid haemorrhages are treated by an interventional coiling procedure undertaken by interventional radiologists.

G. Rebleeding from aneurysms, hydrocephalus and vasospasm are the main immediate complications and may result in rapid neurological deterioration in patients following a subarachnoid haemorrhage.

10

A. The symptoms are suggestive of a muscle disorder. He has features of myotonia (with delayed relaxation of muscles after contraction). The clinical case is compatible with myotonic dystrophy. The condition is characterised by myotonia, wasting of the sternocleidomastoids, dysphagia and muscle weakness.

B. There is an assocation with frontal balding, cataracts, cardiac conduction defects and testicular atrophy.

C. The disease is inherited in an autosomal dominant fashion and usually presents in the third to fourth decades (due to increase in AGC repeats on chromosome 19q13.3).

D. Disease occurs with an earlier age of onset and more severe phenotype in successive generations.

E. Clinical examination, electromyography (EMG changes are found in almost any muscle: waxing and waning of potentials termed the dive bomber effect) and molecular diagnostic testing are all useful.

Index of cases by diagnosis

Neurology: Clinical Cases Uncovered, 1st edition. © M. Macleod,
M. Simpson and S. Pal. Published 2011 by Blackwell Publishing Ltd.

Index

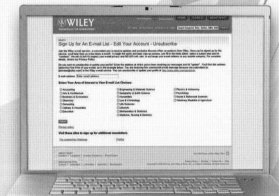
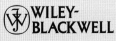

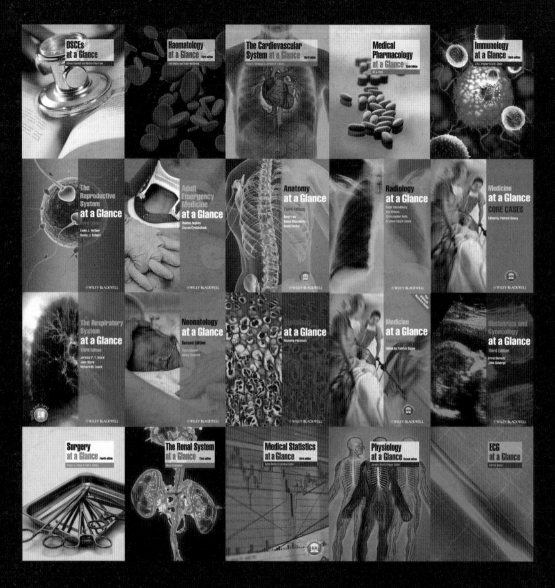
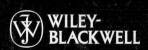